# Management Skills
## for the
## Occupational Therapy Assistant

# Management Skills
### for the
# Occupational Therapy Assistant

*Amy Solomon, OTR*
Quantum Integrations Curriculum and Faculty Development
Denver, Colorado
Montessori School of Denver
Denver, Colorado

*Karen Jacobs, EdD, OTR/L, CPE, FAOTA*
Programs in Occupational Therapy
Boston University
Sargent College of Health and Rehabilitation Services
Boston, Massachusetts

SLACK
INCORPORATED

*An innovative information, education, and management company*
6900 Grove Road • Thorofare, NJ 08086

**www.slackbooks.com**

ISBN: 978-1-55642-538-7

The procedures and practices described in this book should be implemented in a manner consistent with the professional standards set for the circumstances that apply in each specific situation. Every effort has been made to confirm the accuracy of the information presented and to correctly relate generally accepted practices. The authors, editor, and publisher cannot accept responsibility for errors or exclusions or for the outcome of the material presented herein. There is no expressed or implied warranty of this book or information imparted by it. Care has been taken to ensure that drug selection and dosages are in accordance with currently accepted/recommended practice. Due to continuing research, changes in government policy and regulations, and various effects of drug reactions and interactions, it is recommended that the reader carefully review all materials and literature provided for each drug, especially those that are new or not frequently used. Any review or mention of specific companies or products is not intended as an endorsement by the author or publisher.

SLACK Incorporated uses a review process to evaluate submitted material. Prior to publication, educators or clinicians provide important feedback on the content that we publish. We welcome feedback on this work.

Published by:          SLACK Incorporated
                       6900 Grove Road
                       Thorofare, NJ 08086 USA
                       Telephone: 856-848-1000
                       Fax: 856-853-5991
                       www.slackbooks.com

Contact SLACK Incorporated for more information about other books in this field or about the availability of our books from distributors outside the United States.

Library of Congress Cataloging-in-Publication Data

Solomon, Amy, 1955-
  Management skills for the occupational therapy assistant / Amy
Solomon, Karen Jacobs.
      p. ; cm.
  Includes bibliographical references and index.
  ISBN 1-55642-538-4 (pbk.)
  1. Occupational therapy assistants.
  [DNLM: 1. Occupational Therapy--organization & administration. 2.
Office Management.  WB 555 S689m 2003]  I. Jacobs, Karen, 1951- II.
Title.
RM735.4 .S655 2003
615.8'515'068--dc21
                              2002015485

Printed in the United States of America

Last digit is print number: 10  9  8  7

# Dedication

To my Father,
in loving memory of his sensitivity, spirit, and insight and with much thanks
for instilling in me a love of learning and sense of wonder.
And to my Mother,
for her generosity, loving heart, open mind, and perseverance and
whose OT footsteps I have followed.
—Amy


To my family with much love and admiration.
—Karen

# Contents

Instructors: The *Management Skills for the Occupational Therapy Assistant Instructor's Manual* is also available from SLACK Incorporated. Don't miss this important companion to *Management Skills for the Occupational Therapy Assistant*. To obtain the *Instructor's Manual*, please visit http://www.efacultylounge.com

# Acknowledgments

We gratefully acknowledge the expertise of our contributing authors, without whom this text would be far less rich in information. As well, we recognize with much gratitude the assistance and patience of our publisher, SLACK Incorporated. Thank you to John Bond, publisher; Amy McShane, editorial director; Jennifer Stewart, managing editor; Robert Smentek, project editor; and Lauren Plummer, design editor for their unwavering support.

To our families, for their patience and support throughout the completion of this project, we say thank you, with much love.

And to those who have traveled the OT road with us, particularly our students and mentors. We realize, with much appreciation, the contribution you have made to our professional development. Without you, the inspiration for this text might never have come about.

# About the Authors

Amy Solomon, OTR has been an occupational therapist since 1982 when she graduated from Colorado State University with a bachelor of science in occupational therapy. She is currently in the process of completing her thesis for her advanced master's degree in occupational therapy, also from Colorado State. Amy's clinical practice has focused primarily in the area of inpatient psychiatry at Denver Health Medical Center (formerly Denver General Hospital). Her other clinical experience includes inpatient rehabilitation and home health. During her tenure at Denver General Hospital, she became involved in education as the fieldwork coordinator for the OT Department in the Department of Psychiatry. Deciding that education was her passion, she began teaching in the OTA Program at Arapahoe Community College in Littleton, CO in 1994, moving on to develop and direct the OTA Program at Denver Technical College from 1995 through 2001. In July 2003, Amy will begin her second consecutive term on the Roster of Accreditation Evaluators of the Accreditation Council for Occupational Therapy Education of the American Occupational Therapy Association. She recently completed her term as newsletter editor for the Occupational Therapy Association of Colorado. Amy is currently a curriculum writer/developer for Quantum Integrations in Denver and also serves as a lower elementary team member at the Montessori School of Denver.

Karen Jacobs, EdD, OTR/L, CPE, FAOTA is the immediate and past president of the American Occupational Therapy Association. Dr. Jacobs is a professor of occupational therapy at Boston University. She earned a doctoral degree at the University of Massachusetts, a master's at Boston University, and a bachelor's at Washington University in St. Louis, MO.

In addition to being an occupational therapist, Dr. Jacobs is also a board-certified professional ergonomist and the founding editor of the international journal *WORK: A Journal of Prevention, Assessment and Rehabilitation*. Two special areas of research interest are children and backpack use and "healthy computing," as more Americans, children and adults, spend increasing time working at computer keyboards, putting themselves at risk for repetitive strain injuries and other conditions that can result from overuse.

Karen is also an entrepreneur. She is the co-founder of Field Informatics, LLC, a software developer for personal digital assistants (PDAs).

Karen Jacobs has appeared in a number of print and broadcast stories about occupational therapy, including the *New York Times*, *U.S. News and World Report*, *Business Week*, *20/20*, CNN, NPR, and others. She is also the co-host of the Andover local access television show, *Lifestyle by Design*.

# Contributing Authors

Sue Berger, MS, OTR is clinical instructor at Sargent College, Boston University. She also has extensive experience teaching at occupational therapy assistant programs in Massachusetts. She is an RAE for ACOTE and faculty subsection coordinator for EDSIS, Her clinical experience spans the health care continuum, with specific interest in occupational therapy's role with hospice care, individuals with HIV/AIDS and individuals with low-vision living in the community.

Pamela DiPasquale-Lehnerz, MS, OTR has been an occupational therapist since 1978. She received her bachelor of science degree in occupational therapy from Eastern Michigan University and her master of science degree, also in occupational therapy, from Colorado State University. Currently, she is pursuing a doctorate in health services research at the University of Colorado Health Sciences Center. Pamela has extensive clinical experience in physical rehabilitation and has served in numerous supervisory and program manager positions over the last 10 years, including positions on the spinal cord injury team at Craig Rehabilitation Hospital in Denver and the Rehabilitation Institute of Chicago. Pamela is also active within the legislative element in Colorado, serving on the Colorado Division of Workers Compensation Medical Treatment Guidelines for Low Back Pain Task Force and working to pass the Deceptive Trade and Title Protection Act in Colorado, which protects the occupational therapist title. She has served in the Occupational Therapy Association of Colorado since 1981 and is currently the legal/finance chairperson and state liaison to the AOTA State Regulatory Network. Most recently, she has been recognized by her peers by being awarded the Marjorie Ball Award of Merit, the highest award that an OT can receive in the state of Colorado.

Jeffrey D. Hsi received his PhD from the University of Michigan and his JD from Rutgers University School of Law. He practices law in Boston, Massachusetts.

Jennifer Kaldenberg, MSA, OTR/L, CLVT is the director of Occupational Therapy Services New England College of Optometry and New England Eye Institute. She is also a lecturer at New England College of Optometry (Vision Rehabilitation Course).

David L. Lee, MS, OTR/L completed his post-professional master's degree in occupational therapy teaching curriculum at Boston University, Sargent College of Health and Rehabilitation Sciences. Mr. Lee is an occupational therapist at Spaulding Rehabilitation Hospital in Boston, MA, working previously on the spinal cord injury and addictions unit, and now in general areas including upper extremity/musculoskeletal, brain injury, pain, cardiopulmonary, and psychosocial dysfunctions. A consultant in upper extremity disorders and office ergonomics for health care professionals, Mr. Lee has a considerable interest in occupational ergonomics, computer technology, and assistive technology.

Amy Wagenfeld received her PhD from Walden University and her BS in Occupational Therapy from Western Michigan University. She is on the faculty at Lasell College in Newton, MA and is a private occupational therapy consultant.

# Preface

With the demand in health care for practitioners to be more astute in a business sense and conscious of the management and financial issues associated with health care today, it is fitting that the occupational therapy assistant (OTA) be familiarized with administrative functions. In addition, in a fast-paced environment where the business part of practice plays a significant role, clinical decisions must be made with judgment and insight that consider the administrative position. The OTA entering the field will have a leading edge if he or she is able to consider management's role, execute leadership skills, and understand financial, legal, and regulatory obligations.

The goal of this text is to introduce these concepts to the OTA student and motivate the student to think about these issues and incorporate them into their clinical decision-making as they embark on their career. The student will undoubtedly learn more about administration, management, and leadership in the field, as well as become familiar with the specific requirements of their chosen area of practice. The intent of this book is to give students a "jumping off point" from which they can become familiar with these concepts and consolidate them into practice.

# ROLES AND RESPONSIBILITIES OF THE OCCUPATIONAL THERAPY ASSISTANT IN MANAGEMENT

*Amy Solomon, OTR*

## Introduction

As an occupational therapy assistant (OTA) instructor, I have been confronted with the question, "How much training in management should OTA students be given?" The traditional perspective, in general, is that certified occupational therapy assistants (COTAs) are trained to do the hands-on patient care, while occupational therapists who are registered (OTRs) are trained to do the evaluations and administrative functions. In fact, I have been asked by more than one OTA student why they need to learn management and administrative functions when they will be doing patient care.

While in the formal organizational structure the OTR is most likely to have the majority of administrative responsibility, the COTA will be required to take administrative issues, such as legalities and regulatory issues, into consideration when making clinical judgments. In addition, the COTA may be asked to contribute to administrative processes, and to do so effectively, must understand them. Most importantly, in today's health care system, all personnel must use independent clinical judgment, and the COTA must be able to make sound clinical decisions. The importance of administrative issues cannot be underestimated in this decision-making process. Because of the health care environment today, management, administrative, and business issues must be a part of clinical reasoning.

Table 1–1 summarizes the administrative domains that the COTA should understand as a part of practice. Each of these topics is covered in a chapter of this book.

The purpose of this chapter is to provide an overview—the "big picture"—of management and leadership. The descriptions found in this chapter will give the reader a sense of what is expected from those in management and leadership positions, and will give an overview of the context in

Table 1-1

## Administrative and Management Domains

| Administrative/Management Role or Concept | Definition |
| --- | --- |
| Change and the history of occupational therapy | Health care and occupational therapy are continually changing. Knowing where the profession has been and know where it is today can facilitate understanding of administrative and management issues. |
| Credentialing issues, ethics, and legalities | • Credentialing is the awarding of a title to an individual or institution that has met a set of predetermined criteria.<br>• Ethics involve the moral side of practice and meeting the standards identified in the Occupational Therapy Code of Ethics.<br>• Legal concerns are those that are related to the regulation of practice by government agencies. |
| Reimbursement and finance | Largely related to the business aspects of practice, these issues deal with funding, payment of service, and budgets. |
| Staffing requirements and constraints | Staffing refers to the number of staff available to provide treatment and intervention, support staff, and others as applicable to the setting. The OT manager is generally responsible for the OT staff and must balance effective care with productivity standards. |
| Supervision and continued professional development | Supervision is an ongoing process focused on skill and professional development. As an entry-level COTA, your supervisor will work with you to develop practice and other professional skills. |
| Communication | This refers to the ability to interact effectively with all members of the health care team, including administrators. Communication can be enhanced throughout the application of several techniques. Communication skills are as important in management tasks as they are in interacting with patients and clients. |

continued

Table 1–1 continued

## Administrative and Management Domains

| ADMINISTRATIVE/MANAGEMENT ROLE OR CONCEPT | DEFINITION |
|---|---|
| Continuous quality management | The process in which services are continually monitored and evaluated against objective standards to ensure that service needs are met. |
| Research | Research is a systematic and structured acquisition of professional knowledge. Practice activities and intervention supported by research is necessary for credibility, expanding the knowledge base of the profession, and for validating OT to third-party payers. |
| Entrepreneurship | One who is an entrepreneur is one who recognizes business opportunities and takes action to creatively meet them. It is a blend of leadership and creativity executed within professional constraints. |

which the skills discussed in this text occur. Subsequent chapters will focus on the tools that the COTA can utilize in the practice setting to develop entry-level management and leadership skills. As the COTA grows professionally, he or she may desire to further develop these skills in greater depth.

This chapter will also provide an overview of the professional organizations that provide leadership and management to the profession of occupational therapy. Organizations such as the American Occupational Therapy Association (AOTA), the National Board for Certification in Occupational Therapy (NBCOT), the World Federation of Occupational Therapists (WFOT), the American Occupational Therapy Foundation (AOTF), the Accreditation Council for Occupational Therapy Education (ACOTE), and state organizations will be described.

In order to introduce the COTA's involvement in the management process, we will review three major categories: management, leadership, and business. The tasks of administration typically fall into at least one of these categories.

# Management

In everyday professional language, management tends to be viewed as running a department or organization. Here, we will break the task of running a department into three roles: management (task), leadership (how one conducts oneself and responds to others and situations), and business (ensuring the future viability of a department or organization).

Management is the task part of maintaining and developing an occupational therapy (OT) practice. It includes the administrative aspects of running a department or practice

## INTRODUCTORY ACTIVITY—CATEGORIZING MANAGEMENT AND LEADERSHIP TASKS

Using the following list, categorize the tasks as to whether they are management or business related. It is possible (and acceptable) for a task to fall into more than one category.

- Writing or contributing to the development of the OT department budget
- Writing or contributing to a job description
- Participating in interviewing a candidate for a new staff position
- Setting continuing education goals with a new COTA
- Completing an annual performance review with a staff member
- Participating in a quality management study
- Participating in a research study
- Contributing to program development to meet new regulatory guidelines
- Resolving a roles conflict with a physical therapy department
- Documenting your treatment session
- Contributing to the development of a fieldwork program
- Contributing to OT program development
- Following CMS/Medicare guidelines
- Writing or contributing to policy and procedure

and ensures that tasks are completed thoroughly, accurately, and in a timely fashion. Managing an OT setting includes the operational functions of a department and may include the specific tasks defined in Table 1–2.

COTAs may be involved in any of these aspects of management, depending on your state's practice act guidelines, facility policy and accreditation requirements, third-party payer demands, and individual level of experience. Each of these elements, especially in today's health care environment, play a role in clinical decisions regarding prioritizing intervention goals, discharge planning, and making recommendations for continuation of care. Consequently, although the OTR is usually ultimately responsible for management duties, the COTA must take management issues, such as budget constraints and reimbursement, into consideration in daily decision-making. The COTA, who may move in an administrative direction as he or she grows professionally, will require a strong working knowledge of management concerns. The chapters of this text will introduce the foundations of significant management tasks.

## Management Styles

Management styles vary considerably, depending on organizational structure and goals and the manager's personality and experience. The manager's style is a major factor in determining the work climate. A manager's style provides behavioral cues to the people they supervise and sets an example for conduct (Watkins, 1996). Several styles have been defined and will be summarized here. Because an in-depth study of management theory is

Table 1-2

## *Tasks of Occupational Therapy Management*

| MANAGEMENT TASK | DEFINITION |
| --- | --- |
| Staffing | Includes assigning staff in appropriate numbers based on patient/client census, productivity standards, and patient/client needs. Hiring and dismissal may also be part of this responsibility. |
| Budgeting | Determining capital and operational needs based on direct and indirect costs (see Chapter 5). Involves working with upper management to conform to organizational budgeting. |
| Maintaining productivity levels | Ensuring that staff/patient ratios are appropriate to showing a revenue stream from the OT department. |
| Creating and implementing policy and procedure | Writing protocols and rationales for department function; takes into consideration organization and regulatory guidelines. |
| Scheduling patients/clients | Ensuring that patients/clients are seen in a timely manner. Involves prioritizing patients on the bases of acuity, policy, and in collaboration with other scheduling needs. |
| Scheduling staff | Assigning work periods and responsibilities to staff in a manner that supports productivity standards and patient/client needs. With OT services being required 7 days per week in many settings, staff scheduling also involves being sure to equitably rotate staff through weekend hours. |
| Planning and conducting meetings | Facilitating meetings in a manner that effectively, yet efficiently, meets department and organizational goals. Typically involves a weekly OT staff meeting and others as needed for special issues. The OT manager will be involved with meetings outside of the OT department. |
| Providing supervision | Interacting on a regular basis with department members to ensure skill development and professional growth. Involves recognition and disciplinary action as appropriate. Includes completing performance reviews and following up on professional development plans. |

continued

*Table 1-2 continued*

## Tasks of Occupational Therapy Management

| MANAGEMENT TASK | DEFINITION |
|---|---|
| Billing and overseeing billing procedures | Makes sure billing is done accurately and on time; follows up on billing issues. Sees that billing is done in accordance with regulatory stipulations. |
| Ordering and maintaining supplies | Involves maintaining supplies on hand to meet patient/client needs, maintaining communication with treatment staff regarding inventory and needs, knowing timeframes for ordering and delivery, and working within the budget. |
| Ensuring compliance with accreditation and other regulatory bodies | Knowing current state, accreditation, and other regulations so that department operations are in compliance. Involves staying current on regulatory updates and modifying policy and procedure accordingly. |

beyond the scope of this text, the reader interested in pursuing these ideas is referred to the reference list at the close of the chapter. Numerous other resources in printed and electronic formats are available.

Watkins (1996) identifies a *collaborative* management style, versus a *competitive* management style. The collaborative style is characterized by cooperation and respect between departments within an organization, open communication, and a strong emphasis on teamwork. Strong working relationships characterize collaborative management.

The opposite of collaborative management is competitive management, characterized by minimal communication and lack of coordinated efforts between departments. There may be visible contention between departments. Such a style is incompatible with cooperative teamwork (Watkins, 1996).

Blake and Moulton (as cited in Perinchief, 1998; O'Hair et al., 1998) list five management styles.

### THE COUNTRY CLUB STYLE

This approach to management stems from the belief that putting the needs of people first is the primary goal of management. Organizational goals come second to, and may be incompatible with, interpersonal needs. The manager who employs this style is highly supportive and may not make strong demands on workers to meet organizational objectives. The emphasis here is on feelings of well-being among the staff. Use of this style may be appropriate when rapport building is necessary. Its excessive use will undermine productivity concerns and is unrealistic in today's health care environment.

### LAISSEZ-FAIRE MANAGEMENT

This style is characterized by minimal involvement with people or leadership toward organizational goals. In fact, "laissez-faire" is French for "leave you alone." In this style, people are, for the most part, left to function on their own in the status quo. It is the proverbial "bare minimum." There is enough demand here only to maintain minimal standards in terms of productivity and staff morale. This style may be appropriate in situations where process is standardized and there is little room for change. It may be a temporary approach when more pressing concerns demand attention. It is not appropriate in a competitive, rapidly moving environment, such as that found in health care and business today, as it may result in the organization or department falling behind current practice and business developments.

### AUTHORITY–COMPLIANCE OR AUTHORITARIAN MANAGEMENT

The human element and people's needs are given minimal importance (if at all) in this situation. Adhering to productivity and organizational goals are the main focus in this style of management. Efficiency is the primary concern and the work environment is structured in a manner that minimizes the chance that the human element will interfere with production. Because productivity is the bottom line for an organization's survival, this style may be appropriate on a temporary basis to ensure the continuation of an organization. Used regularly, this style may alienate and discourage staff and may result in loss of motivation and commitment.

### PARTICIPATIVE OR TEAM MANAGEMENT

This approach operates on the assumption that if people work toward common organizational goals, then their morale will be raised and an environment of trust and cooperation will ensue. The manager using this style will delegate tasks, and trust that the work will be done. The philosophy is especially effective if workers engage in tasks for which they are intrinsically motivated. Recognition plays an important role in this approach. Generally, this style promotes individual responsibility and self-esteem. The staff must be self-motivated, know their job well, have good judgment, and demonstrate a fair amount of professional maturity for this style to be used consistently in its pure form.

### RULES-ORIENTED MANAGEMENT

This style is characterized by strong managerial control, which is deemed necessary for completion of organizational goals. Enforcement of policy and adherence to procedure are the primary methods of motivating when using this style. A strong emphasis on rules and compliance make this an appropriate method of management when it is necessary to establish order in an organization.

In 1961, Rensis Likert (as cited in O'Hair et al., 1998) described management styles on a continuum with strong emphasis on relationship factors at one extreme and task emphasis on the other. We may envision the continuum as represented in Figure 1–1.

Along the continuum, variations in the task-to-relationship ratio are represented. In other words, some styles emphasize task and relationships equally, while others may lean more heavily toward one or the other. The endpoints of Likert's continuum are the extremes of each.

## Applying Knowledge of Management Styles

There are no definite rules as to whether one should be more relationship oriented, more rules oriented, or more bottom line oriented. Each style has its own merit, depending on the situation. In every situation, priorities and stakeholders are different and will determine the appropriate management task and style. For example, there are situations in which a manager must maintain morale and cohesiveness in a department. A more supportive management style, such as country club or participative, may help achieve this goal. Conversely, in a time of crisis when operational concerns must take first priority and decisions made quickly, a more rules-oriented or authoritarian style may be more appropriate.

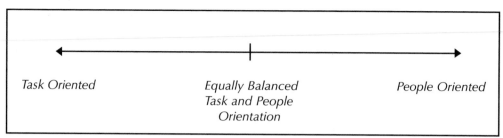

**Figure 1–1.** Conceptualization of Likert's Scale. According to this model, management styles can fall anywhere along this continuum. Although individuals tend to have a tendency toward one end of the scale, it is beneficial to one's management skills to develop all areas and adjust one's emphasis to the needs of the situation.

It is helpful for the entry-level COTA to understand different management styles as they relate to professional socialization and supervision. By having an awareness of different management styles, one can understand why a manager may take certain approaches to different situations. An understanding of how management style plays a part in the administrative process will allow practitioners at any level of experience to understand and play a supportive role in departmental management. For example, assume for a moment that you are now a COTA, and you notice that your manager is not as attentive to interpersonal needs as usual. The manager is assuming a more authoritarian and rigid approach to managing daily productivity and is greatly concerned with efficiency and meeting organizational goals. It would be helpful for the COTA to be aware that the upper management has told your OT manager that a certain level of productivity must be met, or the staff will be required to cut their hours. Since an authoritarian style is more focused on meeting this type of concrete, bottom-line goal, your manager has assumed the style that is most appropriate to the job that needs to be accomplished. When one understands the uses of the different management style, communication and collaboration are made more possible, creating a more positive environment.

An awareness of management styles may also facilitate the supervision process (Chapter 6 covers the supervisory relationship in depth). As a new OT practitioner, you will be applying newly learned skills, as well as becoming familiar with your facility's procedures. Until you become familiar with your new position and its process and procedure, you may feel that you need additional structure and guidance from your supervisor to accomplish daily tasks. In this case, the style of management that focuses on structure and order (such as rules-oriented) will help you learn new procedures as well as increase your confidence in applying familiar ones. As you become more acclimated, this style of supervision may be altered to support you in exploring other goals in accordance with your interests.

In addition, understanding the different styles allows one to understand the style to which they best respond. Understanding what motivates you to learn, develop professionally, as well as be productive will enable you to let your supervisor know your needs in the supervision process.

The reader is reminded that it is unlikely that these styles will appear in "pure" form, as discussed in the previous section. Each person's management style is likely to be a blend of the different styles.

The remaining chapters in this text include skills that will support you in making these judgments.

# Leadership

Traditionally, a leader has been defined as "someone who acts as a guide" (Cayne, 1993, p. 562). Gilkeson (1997) qualifies leaders as those who provide innovation, development, focus on people, utilize trust, and "do the right thing." Leaders "challenge, inspire, enable, model, and encourage," according to Kouzes and Posner (1987, p. 1). Leadership is utilizing "people skills" (Carnegie & Associates, 1993). Bennis and Nanus (1985) state that the definition of leadership changes with the times, but its basic premises remain the same. There are numerous definitions of leadership, as well as a significant amount of literature, all with consistent threads of interacting and working effectively with people, dealing with and adapting to change, and setting example.

At first glance, leadership styles may seem identical to the information used to describe management styles. The literature does distinguish between management and leadership styles and how they are used. While the styles appear similar, leadership differs from management primarily in that management is generally focused on directing people in the accomplishment of daily tasks, while leadership focuses on developing people and the organization over time.

To illustrate the difference between management and leadership, let us create a hypothetical supervision situation. Our supervisees are two COTAs who have been practicing for 2 and 3 years, respectively. Both have become somewhat restless on the job, feeling as though they wish to expand their skills, yet neither is sure of the direction in which to move. The result in the OT department is an atmosphere of sluggishness and low energy that is affecting the function of department. Sensing this, and acknowledging it in supervision, the COTAs' supervisor involves both the COTAs in developing a plan that alters the structure of the daily routine. The goal of this change is to give the COTAs new and additional responsibilities in order to explore some new areas. In doing so, the supervisor considers facility policies, accreditation and licensure requirements, and is careful to approve plans that ensure that daily tasks will be accomplished.

During this period of exploration, one of the COTAs finds that being involved with fieldwork education is a stimulating direction in which to move, and sets goals to expand the student program as well as supervise a fieldwork student. The other COTA decides that program development and quality assurance is the way to go, and sets goals to write new programs for the department, as well as contribute to the quality assurance committee at the hospital. Once the COTAs have set their goals, their supervisor works with them on learning the necessary skills to succeed at their new responsibilities. In doing so, the supervisor employs various management styles. The OT department is once again vibrant, and its staff motivated and excited about their work.

By making this move, the supervisor has recognized and responded to a need for change in the department and devised a way to respond to numerous individual, department, organizational, and regulatory needs. The supervisor has motivated the staff to grow while supporting programming. The vitality of the department has been maintained with innovation and change. This is an example of leadership.

When considering the specifics of the COTA's new responsibilities, the supervisor must manage the tasks and the individuals to see that procedures are carried out in acceptable timeframes and according to protocol. This aspect of the supervisor's job is management. In day-to-day operations, management and leadership may be closely intertwined.

With the accelerated rate of change and exchange of information in today's world, leaders must, more than ever, be looking forward and willing to constantly learn. As health care

changes, the qualities of leadership become more critical to the occupational therapy practitioner. If the reader is interested in reading more about leadership, an exploration of the
literature is recommended. Jacobs (1998) suggests that leadership can be learned through
courses, seminars, on-the-job behavioral training, and mentorship. Here, we will examine
issues that are relevant in current OT practice and explore the qualities of leadership that
can support one's practice and individual development, as well as the profession itself.

## Leaders are Future-Oriented, Innovative, and View Change as Opportunity

When the status quo shows signs of changing, those with leadership characteristics begin
to look for ways in which their organization, department, or profession can adapt to move
with the changes. Rather than mourning the "way things used to be," a leader will look at
what *could* be, given the new set of circumstances. The leader will look at new situations
imaginatively and create possibilities and opportunities in them. Leaders have a vision for
the ideal future and work toward it (Kouzes & Posner, 1987). It is important to recognize,
however, that as leaders create opportunity, they do so with a high regard for values, ethics,
and professional boundaries. For instance, in the changing health care market of the 1990s,
practitioners exercised leadership in recognizing a niche for OT in "non-traditional" areas
of community practice, such as the correctional system, homeless shelters, and numerous
others. These practitioners, however, moved to these new arenas while advocating the values and ethics of OT, as well as supporting OT practice in these settings with a rationale
based in OT theory. This leads to our second premise of leadership.

## Leaders Function With Impeccable Ethics and Integrity

Leaders are said to do the "right thing" (Kouzes & Posner, 1987). A true leader will not
simply forge ahead for the sole purpose of doing something new and notable. A leader's
innovative ideas are based in sound principles of conduct, reflect a respectable mission supported by professional values, and demonstrate a strong regard for colleagues, clients, and
professional boundaries and parameters. Leaders maintain a high regard for regulatory guidelines and standards of quality. While this is not to say that leaders agree with everything,
they demonstrate the ability to address disagreement with respect and assertiveness. They
work toward and contribute to change through acceptable channels, and if change does not
occur, they are able to adapt to get the job done without compromising their basic values.

## Leaders Have a Clear Sense of Their Values, Strengths, and Weaknesses, as Well as a Strong Sense of Direction; In Addition, They Maintain Current Knowledge of Relevant Professional and Organizational Issues

Knowing where one excels, as well as one's boundaries and limits, allows one to know
where he or she stands on issues and what he or she can or cannot accomplish. Combined
with continuous learning, one maintains a perspective on relevant developments and is able
to position oneself and take appropriate action to be effective. From this vantage point, a
leader recognizes growth opportunities and motivates and engages others to act.

# Leaders are Aware of and Sensitive to the Needs of People and Organizations

Leaders honor and respond to the needs of those around them, treating others with consistent ethics and values. Leaders encourage and support innovation in the people with whom they work, motivate them to achieve their goals, and encourage their development. Leaders bring out the best in those with whom they work while supporting the goals of the organization. In times of change, they instill assurance and guidance with innovation and spirit. They also acknowledge the personal and professional accomplishments of their colleagues. Kouzes and Posner (1987) call this "encouraging the heart."

Again, this is not to say that leaders are always happy-go-lucky and believe everything is positive and bright. Leaders see the pitfalls in situations and, at times, must be firm in their stance with others. The significance here is the manner in which they view setbacks and deal with people. Difficulties are viewed from a problem-solving perspective. Colleagues' views are respected, if not agreed with. Mistakes are viewed as learning situations and a leader will work with a colleague to develop him- or herself. The leader will be appropriately confrontive when necessary.

Based on the way they treat others, leaders are able to motivate others to work toward a common goal (Kouzes & Posner,1987).

# Leaders Model Self-Awareness and an Attitude of Personal Development by Learning From Their Mistakes and Achievements

A hallmark of effective leaders is that they model what they strive to motivate in others (Kouzes & Posner, 1987). In order to do this, they must demonstrate the self-awareness and exercise the self-control to remain rational and thoughtful, to model dealing with change, overcoming obstacles, and maintaining and working toward a vision. This is not to say leaders do not feel emotion; indeed, another characteristic of leaders is passion—and this entails emotion—but they know how and when to express it.

# Leaders Acknowledge and Learn From Their Mistakes as Well as From Their Achievements

Leaders do not place blame for their errors; rather, they offer a solution for correcting them. They take lessons from something successful as well and apply it in other circumstances. They recognize others' achievements and give credit where credit is due (Carnegie & Associates, 1993).

Subsequent chapters on communication, professional supervision, change, and entrepreneurship will provide practical strategies in the development of, and introduce opportunities in which to apply leadership skills.

# Leadership Concepts and OT Practice

When one compares management and leadership, one of the differences that one sees is that the tasks of management are frequently ones that are part of a professional job assignment that comes after a specified amount of experience. Leadership skills, on the other hand, are attributes that anyone can exercise at any time, regardless of their "official" position in the organization. Leadership is more an attitude and manner of completing a task, versus the task itself. Any professional, regardless of where he or she may be on the organizational chart, can demonstrate the qualities of leadership in daily operations. Occupational therapy practitioners can add to the profession and their organization by demonstrating leadership skills. Individually, leadership skills are often viewed as maturity and effectiveness.

# Change in Occupational Therapy

Occupational therapy practice is constantly affected by change. Recent changes in Medicare funding have precipitated extensive alterations in reimbursement, resulting in changing staffing patterns and job availability for occupational therapists. In the past, other changes, such as those brought about by the advent of diagnostic-related groups (DRGs) in the early 1980s and reduction in psychiatric services in the mid-1980s have also affected occupational therapy.

## Innovation and Change

In the light of any change, innovation and inspiration permit others to move forward and contribute to a positive environment. One of the impacts of the Balanced Budget Act of 1997 (BBA) was to reduce the number of OT positions in long-term care. One of the innovative responses of some OT personnel was to introduce new programs in "non-traditional" settings. An alternative to mourning "the way things used to be," these practitioners offered new and creative solutions. The process of change will be addressed in Chapter 2 and entrepreneurship (the ability to turn the need for change into opportunity) is covered in Chapter 10.

There are currently some contemporary issues and demands on professionals that call upon leadership skills and offer the OT practitioner opportunities for their application.

## Doing More With Less

As health care dollars become more precious, all practitioners are being requested to be more time-efficient and cost-effective. Upper management actively seeks methods of controlling and reducing costs. While OT personnel must support the business interests of their organization, they must also maintain a strong ethical sense, seeing that intervention is provided by qualified individuals and that patient/client care is appropriate. Cost-efficiency must be strongly balanced with patient/client care and regulatory guidelines. The COTA demonstrates leadership by recognizing and seeking ethical solutions to balancing business and quality issues.

## Continuous Learning and Professional Development

The COTA will be better able to understand current regulatory and ethical issues and offer appropriate innovations if his or her knowledge is current. The leader makes use of professional organizations, publications, and research to stay up-to-date in the field. In addition, the leader is aware of the self and is open to constructive feedback and supervision to continue the process of learning and personal skill development.

# The Leadership Process

As in management, there are different leadership styles, each with its own merits. Recall that leadership (versus management) focuses on people and long-term, large-scale events. Leadership styles are selected based on an outcome that is desired. The styles are similar to those of management in that one may choose what should be prioritized. Liebler, Levine, and Rothman (as cited in Gilkeson, 1997) list five types of leadership styles.

## *Autocratic*

This style of leadership is oriented toward authority, with workers receiving explicit directions with close supervision. Emphasis on individual initiative is minimal. This type of leadership is appropriate in times of crisis when decisions need to be made quickly or when a critical element of the organization is at stake.

## *Bureaucratic*

Similar to the autocratic styles of leadership, the bureaucratic approach is also authority-driven. It differs mainly in that the policies and rules of the organization, which are strictly enforced, form the basis for setting guidelines for goal achievement. Many times, bureaucratic approaches are seen in organizations that are heavy in upper management.

## *Participative*

The participative style of leadership emphasizes the involvement of work teams in the decision-making process. The input of employees and the strengths of individuals are used in the accomplishment of organizational goals. The leader makes final decisions. Participative leadership is appropriate when planning and decision-making are done proactively and buy-in from the work teams is desirable.

## *Laissez-Faire*

This approach to leadership provides minimal to no structure, trusting that individuals are self-motivated and self-directed. Supervision is nominal and the leader functions primarily in a consultant role. This approach is most effective when teams are highly competent and experienced, or when a team will benefit from time to work through its own process.

## *Paternalistic*

The paternalistic leader places little faith in work teams, who are not encouraged to make independent decisions. Rather, they are encouraged and structured in such a way that they become dependent on the leader.

Heifetz (1994) suggests an approach to selecting a leadership style in which an individual considers what is to be achieved, the situations of the people involved, and the general context of the situation at hand. In doing so, an appropriate approach to one's goals can be selected, much as discussed in the management section.

In summary, a leader engages in a complex balancing act. A leader must simultaneously maintain the vision and goals; uphold values; preserve quality of OT services; advocate and uphold ethical, regulatory, and professional boundaries; support and instill motivation in others; and sustain learning and flexibility in order to move forward. In practice, an occupational therapy manager is frequently in a position to balance management tasks, leadership, and business considerations.

# Business Considerations

One of the critical aspects of managing an occupational therapy department is evaluating the cost and benefits of service (Logigian, 1996), as well as balancing sound financial practice with effective service (Perinchief, 1998). Both are important to business concerns, as occupational therapists must support their organizations and render quality and ethical care at the same time.

Rosee (2000) states that, traditionally, OTs have not been an active part of financial management in many instances, as this function was addressed by the business office. She describes a current need for OT managers to broaden their skills to include fiscal management due to changes brought about by the prospective payment system (PPS) in the long-term care setting. In her article, she discusses ways for therapy managers to provide the most effective service under the constraints of PPS.

Although a description of Rosee's strategies is beyond the scope of this text, it is noteworthy to observe the balance for which she strives between business concerns and giving quality care. She states that in achieving this balance, we support the survival of the profession (Rosee, 2000).

Another element of the business aspect of providing OT service is that of organizational planning. Program expansion and goals must be planned and developed in keeping with the organizational goals and vision of top management and, in some programs, consumers (Perinchief, 1998). Departmental planning in the context of the overall organizational development involves assessing the match between department goals and organizational goals, cost and revenue projections, staffing needs, and space and equipment requirements. All of these elements must be considered in conjunction with providing thorough, ethical, and quality care.

Another business consideration in today's health care environment is that of monitoring staffing plans, including justifying staffing by using organizational practice guidelines and accreditation standards and using strategies to reduce staff on a temporary basis as needed (Kurtz, 1999). This provides adequate staffing numbers but allows the manager to reduce staffing when necessary to manage costs.

Other elements affecting business decisions in therapy include the cost of interdisciplinary treatment and how OT fits into the team picture (Kurtz, 1999), as well as federal government constraints, such as those imposed by the Health Care Finance Administration (HFCA), now the Centers for Medicare and Medicaid Services (CMS) (Rosee, 2000).

In summary, OT is in a position to prove itself as cost effective and providing effective and efficient patient/client care at the same time. In doing so, the OT manager must balance quality care with sound business practices. The COTA may be asked to justify or provide rationale for a clinical decision. Understanding, applying, and being able to articulate business considerations add to professional credibility. As these business elements will affect COTA practice, COTAs need to have an ongoing awareness of the issues surrounding them.

# The American Occupational Therapy Association and Professional Organizations

Professional occupational therapy organizations exist worldwide and serve to provide practitioners with resources and information (Niestadt & Crepeau, 1998). The purpose of this section is to describe professional OT organizations and provide a synopsis of their services and purposes. The OTA student is encouraged to become acquainted with their professional organizations and to become members of the American Occupational Therapy Association (AOTA) and their respective state organization. This opportunity provides the student with access to excellent and current professional information, affords professional networking opportunities, and supports the promotion and activity of the profession.

AOTA is the national professional organization for OT practitioners and students in the United States. Other countries also have similar professional organizations for practitioners in each respective nation.

AOTA is an organization whose mission is as follows:

"The American Occupational Therapy Association advances the quality, availability, use, and support of occupational therapy through standard-setting, advocacy, education, and research on behalf of its members and the public" (AOTA, 2002a).

AOTA works to support its members in terms of education and professional development, and promote the profession of occupational therapy through public relations, research, and legislation. Membership in AOTA is voluntary. Because its role is one of an informative and promotional function, it remains separate from any credentialing activities to avoid a conflict of interest. The credentialing aspect is discussed in greater detail in Chapter 4.

The AOTA website (www.aota.org) provides information regarding current legislative actions that affect the field of OT, advances in medical and community health that impact the profession, news releases regarding the field, and related issues. The site also offers articles of information accessible to the general public and information regarding OT and OTA educational programs. The website's "members only" section is a secure area, accessible to AOTA members only, and includes information on professional issues of importance to practitioners. For students, becoming a member of AOTA is an excellent value, and affords numerous resources for research for the nominal cost of student membership. In addition, AOTA has created a career area, accessible on the website, which serves as a resource for both employers seeking occupational therapy personnel and for practitioners researching employment opportunities. To gain better familiarity with the services that AOTA provides, the reader is referred to the AOTA website.

The AOTA also serves as the governing body of the profession and is the vehicle through which members have a voice in the activities of the profession.

## Governing Structures of AOTA

The primary governing and policy-making body of AOTA is the Representative Assembly (RA). It is considered to be the vehicle of AOTA through which members have say in the actions of the organization (AOTA, 2002b).

The RA functions in many ways like the Congress of the United States (AOTA, 2002b) in that:

- It has representatives from each state, proportionate to the state's OT practitioner population
- Representatives debate and vote on issues that are brought to them by committees and members of AOTA
- Representatives are nominated and voted on by colleagues in their own states

Representatives of the RA are elected to a 3-year term and may be re-elected for an additional term. Officers include the speaker, who presides over meetings; the vice-speaker, who serves in the absence of the speaker; and the recorder, who functions as a scribe. There are appointed positions of parliamentarian and sergeant-at-arms, which clarify procedures and disseminate written materials during meetings, respectively. The RA meets once a year for 3 to 4 days prior to the annual AOTA national conference (AOTA, 2000).

## Commissions and Committees of AOTA

Three standing commissions and six standing committees are part of the RA. The three commissions are the Commission on Practice (COP), Commission on Education (COE), and Commission on Standards and Ethics (SEC). Standing committees include Agenda, Bylaws, Policies and Procedures, Credentials Review and Accountability, Nominating, Recognitions, and Strategic Planning.

To have your input into the RA, AOTA suggests getting involved by getting to know your state representative, maintaining current knowledge of activity in the field, and giving input to your representative throughout the year.

Other groups within AOTA include:

### THE ASSEMBLY OF STUDENT DELEGATES

The Assembly of Student Delegates (ASD) consists of the student members of AOTA. Each OT and OTA education program has the opportunity to elect a representative to ASD. ASD meets annually before the national AOTA conference (AOTA, 2002c).

### THE AOTA BOARD OF DIRECTORS

The Board of Directors consists of:
- AOTA officers (president, vice-president, secretary, treasurer, and treasurer-elect)
- Vice-speaker
- Chairperson, committee state association presidents
- The World Federation of OT (WFOT) delegate
- Chairperson, Commission on Practice
- Chairperson, Commission on Education
- Chairperson, Commission on Standards and Ethics
- Chairperson, Special Interest Section (SIS) Steering Committee
- OTA representative to the board

Non-voting members of the Board include:
- AOTA executive director
- President of the American Occupational Therapy Foundation (AOTF)
- ASD representative

Invited participants include:
- A consumer representative
- The American Occupational Therapy Political Action Committee (AOTPAC) chairperson
- Accreditation Council for Occupational Therapy Education (ACOTE) chairperson
- AOTF executive director (AOTA, 2002b)

The AOTA Board of Directors is responsible for the long-term planning for the Association and is responsible for areas such as marketing and public policy, fiscal and budget considerations, and strategic planning.

## THE ACCREDITATION COUNCIL FOR OCCUPATIONAL THERAPY EDUCATION

The Accreditation Council for Occupational Therapy Education (ACOTE) is responsible for maintaining and updating accreditation standards for academic programs and for monitoring accreditation compliance of education programs. ACOTE publishes standards (a set for OT programs and one for OTA programs) against which all educational programs are evaluated.

### THE ROSTER OF ACCREDITATION EVALUATORS

This consists of volunteer educators and practitioners who have been trained in the accreditation evaluative process and who, with a member of ACOTE, evaluate the academic programs through a series of paper reviews and an on-site visit.

## *Publications and Documents of AOTA*

AOTA publishes *The American Journal of Occupational Therapy* (AJOT) and *OT Practice*. AJOT is a journal focused on practice research and papers, and is published on a bimonthly basis. *OT Practice* focuses on non-research articles that are relevant to everyday practice in numerous settings. All publications are a benefit of AOTA membership for practitioners. Student membership includes *AJOT* and on-line access to *OT Practice*. Students have the option of purchasing *OT Practice* for a nominal fee.

AOTA has responded to specialized practice needs in the profession by creating the Special Interest Section (SIS). Each SIS focuses on a specialized area of practice, defined by disability, age, performance areas, or practice settings (AOTA, 2002c). The student is referred to the AOTA website as referenced for a description of each of the Special Interest Sections.

AOTA members may subscribe to as many of the Special Interest Sections as they wish, at a nominal fee for each. Subscribers receive a quarterly newsletter, as well as have access to listervs and specialized areas of the AOTA website. Special Interest Sections are an affordable and effective way to stay updated in your area of practice, or to learn more about other areas of service delivery.

The AOTA also publishes statements and viewpoints in a series of official documents. Some examples of these are the OT Code of Ethics, Standards of Practice, and Uniform Terminology (AOTA, 1996). A selection of some the official AOTA documents is summarized in Table 1–3. The reader is referred to the AOTA publication *Official Documents of the American Occupational Therapy Association* for the complete collection of documents and for further detail of those listed here. The entry-level practitioner (and all practitioners) is encouraged to use these as working documents and a guide to practice whenever questions arise.

## *National Board for Certification in Occupational Therapy*

The National Board for Certification in Occupational Therapy (NBCOT) is charged with ensuring that competent practitioners enter the field of occupational therapy. One of the primary responsibilities of NBCOT is creating and monitoring the certification examinations for the COTA and OTR, thus maintaining the standards for obtaining the credential COTA or OTR. One cannot legally use the credential "COTA" or "OTR" without successfully completing the NBCOT exam and maintaining an updated credential by fulfilling certain requirements. Re-certification as a COTA or OTR is due every 3 years. To qualify

Table 1-3

## Selected Official Documents of the AOTA

| DOCUMENT | DESCRIPTION |
|---|---|
| Incorporation papers and bylaws | These are documents regarding the incorporation of AOTA, the bylaws governing the association, and the interpretation of the bylaws. |
| Accreditation documents | Contains the Standards for an Accredited Educational Program for the Occupational Therapist and Occupational Therapy Assistant. These are the standards by which all educational programs are evaluated. |
| The Occupational Therapy Code of Ethics | This document defines the ethical standards under which all OT practitioners are expected to practice. |
| Core Values and Attitudes of Occupational Therapy Practice | States the values held by the profession; the core values are those that the profession strives to uphold in service delivery and in the causes we promote. |
| Standards of Practice | Defines the *minimal* standards that occupational therapy personnel are expected to meet in practice. |
| Position papers | Written on a variety of subjects, these articulate the association's stance on numerous issues. |
| Roles and functions papers | These statements describe roles of occupational therapy personnel in different settings. |
| Guidelines | Includes guiding principles for documentation practices and supervision. |
| Uniform Terminology | This document lists and defines terminology common across the profession. It is intended to standardize meanings to facilitate communication. |
| Statements | This set of documents promotes OT as a viable discipline for providing intervention in a number of clinical situations. Documents define OT and provide examples of services, emphasizing their efficacy. |
| Knowledge and skills papers | These define specialized skills needed in certain areas of OT practice. |

Adapted from American Occupational Therapy Association (1996). *Official documents of the American Occupational Therapy Association*. Bethesda, MD: Author

for re-certification, a practitioner must complete 36 professional development units over the 3-year period and pay the required fee ($50.00 as of this writing).

NBCOT's continuing competency program outlines the activities that are acceptable as continuing competency activities. These include workshops and conferences, formal academic classes, making professional presentations, publishing, participating in study groups, and others (NBCOT, 2002a) In addition, NBCOT controls the use of the credentials and has the authority to restrict one's right to practice in the event that ethical or practice standards are violated. This is discussed in further detail in Chapter 4. NBCOT maintains records of practitioners' certification status (active or inactive) and provides this information to employers and consumers upon request (NBCOT, 2002b).

NBCOT's website, www.nbcot.org, offers information regarding certification examination registration, review materials, and activities of NBCOT.

## The American Occupational Therapy Foundation

The American Occupational Therapy Foundation (AOTF) develops and provides resources for education and research in occupational therapy. Grants for research and scholarships for studying occupational therapy are available through the foundation (AOTF, 2002a). The foundation publishes *OTJR: Occupation, Participation, and Health* (formerly *The Occupational Therapy Journal of Research*) (AOTF, 2002b). For more information about AOTF, the reader is directed to www.aotf.org.

## The World Federation of Occupational Therapists

The World Federation of Occupational Therapists (WFOT) is an international organization consisting of occupational therapy member organizations from all over the world and representatives from each participating country. Membership is available through AOTA, or one's national organization. WFOT serves as the official international organization for the promotion of occupational therapy. It has been in existence since 1952 and currently has 57 member associations (WFOT, 2001). WFOT's official publication is the *WFOT Bulletin*, and the group can be found on the Internet at www.wfot.org.au.

## State Organizations

In the United States, each state has an occupational therapy association whose purpose is to promote the interests of occupational therapy practitioners within their respective states. Each state organization consists of a governing board of officers, a membership, and delegates to the AOTA representative assembly. Some of the tasks that state organizations may assume include lobbying for and obtaining regulation (for example, passing a practice act for licensure) of occupational therapy practice, advocating OT services in the public and private sectors, and supporting other legislation and issues that affect the practice of occupational therapy at the state level. Individual state associations can be accessed and contacted through the AOTA website, www.aota.org.

The organizations working in the interest of the occupational therapy profession offer the student and practitioner a wealth of information and support. In addition, they provide the opportunity to become involved with the development of OT and to take leadership roles. The information presented here is an overview of the activities and services that these organizations supply to their members. As students and entry-level COTAs, you are invited and encouraged to get involved.

# Summary

This chapter has focused on the roles management and leadership in occupational therapy and presented ways in which the COTA can conceptualize both management and leadership. A major theme in the chapter is that COTAs, although not typically department managers, must understand and apply management, leadership, and business principles in their clinical reasoning and daily activities. The remainder of this text is directed at the development of skills to carry out management, leadership, and business functions.

The chapter also summarized major organizations of the occupational therapy profession. Students are encouraged to maintain membership in their national and state associations, utilize the resources they offer to remain current on issues facing occupational therapy as a profession, and be active at the organizational level.

# References

American Occupational Therapy Association. (1996). *Official Documents of the American Occupational Therapy Association*. Bethesda, MD: Author.

American Occupational Therapy Association. (2002a). *About us*. Retrieved November 4, 2002, from www.aota.org/general/about.asp

American Occupational Therapy Association. (2002b). *AOTA Governance*. Retrieved November 4, 2002, from www.aota.org/members/area6/index.asp

American Occupational Therapy Association. (2002c). *Students*. Retrieved November 4, 2002, from www.aota.org/featured/area2/index.asp

American Occupational Therapy Association. (1996). *Official documents of the American Occupational Therapy Association*. Bethesda, MD: Author.

American Occupational Therapy Foundation. (2002a). *Mission, vision, and goals*. Retrieved November 13, 2002, from www.aotf.org/html/mission.html.

American Occupational Therapy Foundation. (2002b). *Facts about the American Occupational Therapy Foundation*. Retrieved November 13, 2002, from www.aotf.org/html/facts.html.

Bennis, W., & Nanus, B. (1985). *Leaders: The strategies for taking charge*. New York: Harper and Row.

Cayne, B. S. (1993). *The new Lexicon Webster's dictionary of the English language*. Danbury, CT: Lexicon.

Dale Carnegie & Associates. (1993). *The leader in you*. New York: Author.

Gilkeson, G. E. (1997). *Occupational therapy leadership: Marketing yourself, your profession, and your organization*. Philadelphia: F. A. Davis.

Heifetz, R. A. (1994). *Leadership without easy answers*. Cambridge, MA: The Belknap Press of Harvard University Press.

Jacobs, K. (1998, Nov. 5). The art of negotiation. *OT Week*.

Kouzes, J. M., & Posner, B. Z (1987). *The Leadership Challenge*. San Francisco: Jossey-Bass.

Kurtz, L. A. (1999). Creating realistic productivity standards. *OT Practice, 4*(4), 26-31.

National Board for Certification in Occupational Therapy (2002a) *Certification renewal requirements approved by NBCOT board of directors*. Retrieved November 4, 2002, from http://www.nbcot.org/nbcot/scripts/news_and_events/press_detail_031902.asp.

O'Hair, D., Friedrich, G. W., & Shaver, L. D. (1998). *Strategic communication in business and the professions* (3rd ed.). New York: Houghton-Mifflin.

Perinchief, J. M. (1998). Management of occupational therapy services. In M .E. Neistadt & E. B. Crepeau (Eds.), *Willard and Spackman's occupational therapy* (9th ed.). Philadelphia: Lippincott.

Rosee, M. (2000). The therapist as a fiscal manager: surviving the SNF PPS and Beyond. *OT Practice*, 5(9), 21-26.

Watkins, R. A. (1996). Management styles, structures and roles. In AOTA (Ed.), *The occupational therapy manager*. Bethesda, MD: AOTA.

World Federation of Occupational Therapists. (2001). *Home page*. Retrieved November 4, 2002, from www.wfot.org.au

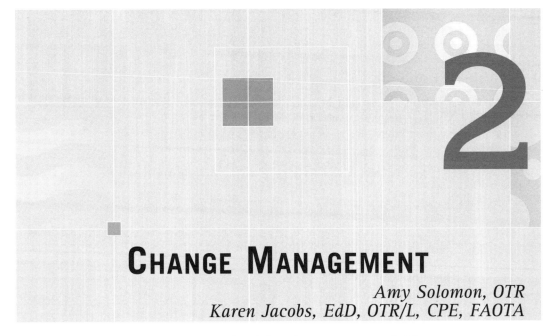

# CHANGE MANAGEMENT

*Amy Solomon, OTR*
*Karen Jacobs, EdD, OTR/L, CPE, FAOTA*

"Organizations that fail to change are sure to fail."
*Robert Kreitner, 1995*

## Introduction

All of us have experienced change to some extent in our lives. There is an old saying that the only thing we can consistently count on is the fact that things will change. In today's world, this is especially true for the occupational therapy manager, who must see departments through periods of change.

Change management involves contending with numerous elements. Practical needs must be addressed, especially in health care, where change can involve modified regulations and requirements that must be implemented into daily procedures. There is the "task" component. Additionally, there are other aspects of change, many involved with interpersonal dynamics. These involve communicating change elements, preparing individuals for change, addressing emotional reactions to change, dealing with resistance, and including people in the change process.

The purpose of this chapter is to examine change, address some of the issues unique to occupational therapy, and explore strategies that individuals and occupational therapy (OT) departments can use in adapting to change.

## Skills You Will Apply

### *Leadership*

A recurring theme throughout this chapter will be that of looking ahead and seeing the possibilities in change. Maintaining an ethical stance and holding one's values are also critical in the change process. Recall that these are characteristic of leadership behaviors. We will discuss others as the chapter progresses.

## *Emotional Competence*

Another recurring theme will be understanding people, recognizing their needs and emotional states, and responding accordingly. Goleman's principles of emotional competence discussed in Chapter 7 are quite applicable in times of change.

# Change in Today's World

The following are characteristics of today's world (Pritchett, 1994):

- Careers are constantly in motion and changing.
- Organizations are continually reshaping themselves.
- The marketplace demands more of organizations, and organizations demand more from employees.
- Organizations and employees must accelerate their pace.
- Priorities and expectations shift, causing ambiguity. Dealing with this involves having a clear role for yourself.
- To succeed in today's world, one needs to take the responsibility to act like a business owner.
- Lifelong learning is the only way to stay competitive in today's changing market.
- Be accountable and contribute more than you cost (add value).
- Be responsible for your own motivation and morale.
- Practice constant quality and improvement personally and related to your organization.
- Be a problem solver.
- Keep an open mind and use change to your benefit.

The elements of leadership are critical to change and perhaps more so than skills of management (Nickols, 2000). From the list above, it is clear that a forward-looking frame of mind, a strong sense of self, and other skills discussed in Chapter 1 contribute to the change process. Looking ahead to Chapter 3, we see that change in the field of occupational therapy is not new, nor is it going to diminish anytime soon. In fact, change can be expected to accelerate.

Technology and the development of communication and information delivery systems have greatly contributed to the rate of change in today's world. This exchange of information has accelerated the manner in which information is exchanged and the rate at which individuals and organizations must respond (Pritchett, 1994). An example is the writing of this text, with contributors from across the United States, co-edited by individuals in Boston and Denver, and published in New Jersey. All of this was accomplished electronically.

Another aspect of communication that warrants consideration is the rate at which information is generated. The complexity of the modern world has created increasingly intricate knowledge in many areas of life. This generation of knowledge perpetuates change and requires that people remain informed and act as necessary in response. Advances in the field of medicine serve as examples.

Change in the field of occupational therapy is also occurring at a significant rate. Advances in technology have allowed occupational therapy practitioners to incorporate computerized solutions into their interventions. Medical science and the impact it has had on individuals' lives and survival has impacted the way in which we deliver treatment. From an administrative perspective, and as described in Chapter 3, political and social change greatly influence our practice.

Change is something to expect in today's world—both in occupational therapy and in a more general sense.

# Responses to Change

Although change is something to be expected, individual reactions to change can vary considerably. Understanding others' reaction to change can provide insight into how to facilitate adaptation to it.

Kreitner (1995) suggests that people will respond to change differently based on whether they perceive the change as something they like or something they dislike. Table 2–1 summarizes this perspective on reactions to change and suggests appropriate leadership in each case.

Another way to assess individual reaction to change is by their locus of control (Moorhead & Griffin, 1989). Individuals with an internal locus of control are likely to want a voice in the change, while those with an external locus of control may withdraw from participating in any related decisions. Leadership should honor these needs as much as possible within the context of the change.

Argyris (as cited in Moorhead & Griffin, 1989) describes a model in which individuals respond to change based on their level of maturity, which tends to increase with work experience. He summarizes seven traits on a continuum from immature to mature, suggesting that individuals with more job maturity respond to change more actively, more independently, with a longer-term perspective and more self-awareness. These traits influence the way in which one responds to change and how they support and lead others in the process.

Individuals may also respond to any life change as a loss, and grief reactions can be observed in situations other than death. When encountering change, one might experience the grief stages of denial, anger, depression, bargaining, and acceptance (Adams & Jones, 1989).

Resistance is a typical response to change (Kreitner, 1995) and occurs for numerous reasons. These may include a sense of loss, issues of trust in management, fear (of losing a job or fear in general), timing of change, personality conflicts with management, lack of tact on the part of management, and disruption to work relationships. Kreitner emphasizes the need to address resistance and suggests education involving individuals as appropriate, supporting, negotiating as possible, providing information in appropriate amounts and with thoughtful timing, and taking actions with the same considerations of tact and timing.

## *Preparing For and Responding To Change*

Nickols (2000) summarizes the change process as a problem-solving process and suggests viewing change as figuring out how to move from one state to another. Skills that should be developed and applied in the problem-solving process include political awareness, analytical skills, interpersonal and communication skills, a knowledge of business, and understanding your organizational system.

Table 2–1

## Kreitner's Model of Reaction to Change

| INDIVIDUAL PERCEPTION | INDIVIDUAL RESPONSE | LEADERSHIP SUGGESTIONS |
| --- | --- | --- |
| Change is something that is perceived as positive | • Initial response may be unrealistic optimism<br>• Over time, reality shock sets in<br>• With time, a more middle ground and constructive participation in the change emerge | The reality shock phase occurs when individuals give up, demonstrate an attitude decline, or have low morale. It is at this stage that leadership becomes critical to see the change through. |
| Change is something that is perceived as negative | • Initial unsureness, trepidation, feelings of being overwhelmed, which may contribute to "getting off on the wrong foot"<br>• Next, an attitude of "blowing it off" or joking about the proposed change tend to follow<br>• When the change continues to occur, the joking stops and individual self-doubt and uncertainty may set in<br>• Then, buy-in begins to occur, possibly after a turning point (e.g., working with supervision, warning, or reprimand)<br>• Lastly, constructive participation occurs | Strong leadership and interpersonal skills will be of value in the middle stages of this situation. An individual must be allowed to vent their feelings, although productivity cannot suffer. In the extreme, the leader may need to assume an authoritarian approach if compliance becomes prolematic. Support for implementing new behaviors in response to change is crucial as well. |

Adapted from Kreitner, R. (1995). *Management* (6th ed.). Boston: Houghton Mifflin.

Strategies to manage change require effective transition management. Moorhead and Griffin (1989) emphasize careful planning and organization as part of transition management, and that daily business must continue during the change process. They articulate the need for managers to take on the role of transition manager in addition to regular management roles and suggest an alternative as assigning an interim manager during the change process.

Bennis, Benne, and Chin (as cited in Nickols, 2000) offer four change-management strategies based on people's characteristics. The four approaches are summarized in Table 2–2.

Table 2-2

## Strategies for Change Management

| STRATEGY | ASSUMPTIONS ABOUT PEOPLE | FACILITATING CHANGE |
|---|---|---|
| Rational–Empirical | People are rational. They will do what is best for them if benefits are pointed out. | Change is successfully implemented when information is communicated and incentives are offered. |
| Normative–Re-educative | People have primarily social interests and it is important for them to follow cultural norms and expectations. | For successful change, redefine and re-interpret existing values and norms while developing a commitment to them. |
| Power–Coercive | People are compliant and and will do what they are told. | Change is implemented when authority is exercised and sanctions are put into place. |
| Environmental–Adaptive | People may not like the disruption brought about by the change, but they will gradually adapt. | Change is successful when implemented over time and people are gradually moved into the new organization. |

Adapted from Nickols, F. (2000). *Change management 101: A primer.* Retrieved September 4, 2002, from http://home.att.net/~nickols/change.htm

As with leadership, there is no one approach that works in all circumstances. This is also true when choosing management and leadership strategies. Nickols (2000) recommends considering the following when selecting a change a management strategy:

- *Degree of resistance*: If resistance is strong, Nickols suggests gradual change (environmental–adaptive), or in some cases, a strong authoritarian approach (power–coercive).
- *People, or target population*: Because there are many different types of people in organizations, a mix of all styles based on needs of the different individuals involved, used judiciously, is probably most effective.
- *What is at stake*: Again, use a blend of all styles to meet as many needs as possible. An intervening variable is what the people involved in the change feel they have to lose.
- *Timeframes*: Emergent situations may call for a power–coercive approach in the interest of getting things done. A less pressing timeframe will allow for the more leisurely style of the other approaches.
- *Expertise of the manager*: With more experience and expertise regarding change available, a manager may use a greater variety of approaches successfully. With less experience, people tend to use the power–coercive approach.

- *Dependency*: According to the extent that management and employees depend on one another, negotiation is a viable option. In other words, in many cases, management cannot function without employees and vice-versa. Therefore, negotiation is appropriate to meet mutual needs.

# Creative Thinking and Change

Traditional approaches to creative thinking, such as brainstorming and problem-solving, can be effectively used in addressing the issues of change. As occupational therapy practitioners, we have a unique edge as a profession.

As a field known for adaptation, occupational therapists are prime candidates for responding creatively to change. Knowledge of activity analysis and adaptation of environments can be applied to processes and organizational change. Here, we will apply our unique perspective as occupational therapists to a change situation.

Occupational therapy training provides the skill of looking at a task or situation, analyzing it for the performance skills that are needed, and deciding what is lacking. In looking at change, the same principles can be applied, taking into consideration the people, the environment, and the tasks at hand. We can see what is needed. Our understanding of task skills, interpersonal and group dynamics, and social-emotional performance can provide great insight in this area. Once we see what is needed from these multiple perspectives, we know how to adapt and fit solutions to the situation.

# Summary

In this chapter, we have considered several aspects of change. We examined change in today's world and how it is characterized by certain demands and needs. Part of change is the rapid delivery of information due to expanding technology. Leadership skills are of significant importance in managing change.

In terms of managing the change process itself, we identified typical responses to change and ways in which leadership might intervene as needed. Responses to change vary, as should leadership's responses, based on the situation. Individual needs, such as perception of change, personal traits, and the situation should all be considered.

Finally, we examined overall models of change, identifying which are appropriate in different situations. Creative thinking has a place in change management, and OT skills can facilitate our involvement in the change process.

# References

Adams, C. H., & Jones, P. D. (1989). *Interpersonal skills and health professional issues.* New York: Glencoe/McGraw-Hill.

Kreitner, R. (1995). *Management* (6th ed.). Boston: Houghton Mifflin.

Moorhead, G., & Griffin, R. W. (1989). *Organizational behavior* (2nd ed.). Boston: Houghton Mifflin.

Nickols, F. (2000). *Change management 101: A primer.* Retrieved September 4, 2002, from http://home.att.net/~nickols/change.htm

Pritchett, P. (1994). *New work habits for a radically changing world: 13 ground rules for job success in the information age.* Dallas: Pritchett & Associates.

# THE HISTORY OF
# HEALTH CARE MANAGEMENT

*Amy Solomon, OTR*

## Introduction

When one reviews the development of health care, one sees a history of legislation that has impacted the delivery of service over the course of time. A further analysis of this history tells us that practitioners over the years have had to demonstrate continuous adaptation to the regulatory environment of the health care professions. As they are today, decisions made in response to changing demographics, health needs, and costs of service provision have had their influence on how and where occupational therapy practitioners provide service. The purpose of this chapter is not so much to provide an extensive and detailed account of historical dates and events, but rather, to summarize the major events of health care evolution that have brought occupational therapy (OT) practice to where it is today.

Jacobs (1996) contributed a chapter to the book *The Occupational Therapy Manager*, published by the American Occupational Therapy Association (AOTA), providing a detailed and thorough history of the development of the current health care environment. The information contained in this resource includes information on the allocation of health care dollars, types of health care organizations, and details of specific health care delivery systems in the United States. It is an excellent resource for the reader who seeks additional detail. The information from Jacobs' chapter has been adapted for the purpose of providing the reader with a synopsis of how we have arrived at out current position.

The history provided in this chapter provides the "big picture" in terms of legislation and social attitudes, and their effect on health care. Chapter 5 (Reimbursement and Finance) will provide the reader with the implications of health care evolution on practice, documentation, lengths of stay, and other aspects of practice.

# Skills You Will Apply

## Management

The tasks of managing an occupational therapy department, such as managing finances and reimbursement issues and ensuring compliance with regulatory guidelines, are directly affected by the activities of the legislature, government offices, and other regulatory bodies. When change occurs, it is not unusual to observe resistance and some of the other emotional reactions described in Chapter 2. While these responses are typical, business must proceed. Understanding the continuous nature of the changing health care arena by examining its history will put current change in perspective. This information also helps the practitioner understand why some regulations are in place and the nature of their intended purpose.

## Leadership

One way in which occupational therapy practitioners demonstrate leadership is to take part in the legislative process as an advocate for the profession, writing letters as a constituent of their congressperson, or becoming involved with the political activities of AOTA. Understanding the legacy of how legislation affects practice will provide a foundation for the practitioner who chooses to become involved in these activities.

## Change

By understanding the context in which these regulations have evolved, we can better appreciate the changes that occur. If we know what has happened in the past and we know how we have arrived at our current position, we can focus on working proactively to move toward those things we desire for our profession and for our individual professional development.

# Where We Are Today

In order to understand where we have been, it sometimes helps to look at where we are, as well as where we are going. As we shall see in this account of the influences that have shaped the administrative and financial aspects of practice, health care has seen constant change. Occupational therapists who have been practicing over the last 20 years have seen major transformation in the way we provide services, the way in which facilities are reimbursed for service, and in practice settings. Change will continue as we move deeper into the 21st century.

Baum (1997) forecasts:

- A community model of health care
- Managed/planned health care
- A focus on prevention, wellness, well-being, and function
- A focus on the environmental context
- An emphasis on individual responsibility
- A community-centered, collaborative (versus competitive), networked health care system

The AOTA, in formulating its long-term strategic plan, projected what OT will be like in the year 2010 and the resources we need to develop to get there. They generated themes addressing holistic approaches, wellness, entrepreneurial opportunities, scientific inquiry, and social consciousness and commitment (AOTA, 1999).

In some ways, we can recognize these elements in the managed systems of today. Conversely, there are those who would say we still making progress in some of these areas. Peloquin (1998) refers to the conflict that exists between cost-effective and efficient business practices and the way in which we provide services. Both of the above perspectives are probably true to some extent.

# A Condensed History

A concern with the humanistic aspects of health care, and its status as a human right, is not new. Historically, it is mentioned in the 1796 Congressional Record, and Franklin Delano Roosevelt alluded to it in 1944.

Government involvement with health care is not new either. Prior to World War II, hospital construction was minimal. In 1947, The Hospital Survey and Construction Act of 1946, Title VI of the Public Health Service Act (more commonly known as and typically referred to as the Hill-Burton Act) evaluated states' needs for hospitals and provided funding for their construction. This recognition of needs and proliferation of hospitals may have been due, in part, to the end of World War II and the needs of returning military personnel.

At various times throughout subsequent decades and into the 1980s, funding from the Hill-Burton Act was expanded in the Mental Retardation Facilities Construction Act (1963 to 1980) and the Community Mental Health Centers Act (1963 to 1980) (Jacobs, 1996).

The effects of additional construction, needed for modernizing facilities as technology advanced, and inflation resulted in a need to control costs and address personnel shortages.

To respond to these developments, additional legislation to promote and support individuals going into health care was enacted. Among these were the Health Amendment Act of 1956, which provided grants to schools of public health and supported the training of public health nurses and personnel; the Nurses' Training Act (1964) and the Health Education Assistance Amendment (1965), which provided money for health professional training; and the Allied Health Professional Personnel Training Act (1966), the first legislation to include occupational therapy in funding. Funding of this nature continued until government support decreased in the late 1970s and 1980s (Jacobs, 1996). Health professional shortages came next, and costs began to increase.

The government became aware of rising expenditures, and attempts to control costs were made. In 1972, an amendment to the Social Security Act created Professional Standards Review Organizations (PSROs). A PSRO consisted of a group of physicians from a specified geographic area and who were charged with monitoring care and costs through utilization review committees.

In 1972, Limitations to Medicare Part A were passed. The National Health Planning and Resources Development Act mandated the creation of a national health care plan and the formation of administrative agencies to ensure effective plans on the state level (Jacobs, 1996).

In 1982, the Tax Equity and Fiscal Responsibility Act (TEFRA) extended the limits on Medicare originally passed in 1972. The limits included OT and other allied health disciplines. In 1983, the Social Security amendments mandated an alteration in funding for health care, which resulted in the diagnostic-related groups (DRGs—explained in greater detail in Chapter 5). DRGs are guidelines that set limits on payment for services, depending on factors such as diagnosis, age, gender, co-existing health concerns, and other demographic considerations. DRGs were implemented on a national basis, affecting acute settings for adult patients. The 1983 legislation also created the Health Care Finance Administration (HCFA), and the implementation of DRGs was the first of the prospective payment system (PPS). Prospective pay means that a predetermined amount of money is set aside for care, rather than retrospective payment, which pays after the fact for any service deemed necessary. Under the DRGs, if a hospital did not spend its entire allocation for a given case, the institution was permitted to keep the difference. Therefore, there was an incentive to keep lengths of stay short and to provide only the most necessary of services of those authorized under the DRGs.

As a result of limitations on inpatient care, there was a need to develop alternatives to traditional hospital care. The outcome was an increase in community and outpatient services, which was also supported by advances in technology, which allowed patients to safely leave the inpatient setting.

To cover these outpatient and community services, funding for Medicare Part B (the part of Medicare that covers services outside of the acute hospital services) was expanded. Increased coverage for skilled nursing facilities (SNFs), rehabilitation hospitals, outpatient facilities, and home health was available. A significant portion of OT service delivery moved to these arenas.

As services moved to these settings, requirements for SNF standards were imposed with the passage of the Omnibus Budget Reconciliation Act (OBRA) of 1987. Among the regulations established by OBRA were requirements for programming content, programs to reduce the use of physical and chemical restraints, standards for the living environment, standards for patients' rights, and guidelines for planning, implementing, and documenting care (Robnett, 1999).

Most recently, the Balanced Budget Act (BBA) of 1997 brought PPS to long-term care facilities, significantly limiting reimbursement for rehabilitation services. Again, the details of how this affects financial aspects of care are discussed in Chapter 5. The result of the BBA for occupational therapists was a significant limitation in the number of hours for service, which affected the job market. Occupational therapists began to move to more community-based settings, such as schools. As a result, with some practicing strong entrepreneurial skills, they responded to change and marketed OT into new settings.

As of this writing, the market is regaining some of the ground it lost to BBA. Occupational therapists are finding a niche in numerous community areas, such as the prison system, home modification, industry, and programs for the homeless (Stancliff, 1997). OTs are moving into new areas where a focus on an individual's occupational performance is a sound intervention. In this way, we are creating the opportunity to validate occupation as sound intervention. Thus, our history will continue to unfold.

# The Effects of Legislation

If we evaluate the historical account above, we see a recurring theme emerging in the sense that when a need or concern arises, an action is taken to fill the need or ameliorate the concern. The action generates new opportunities, which attract practitioners and result in growth in the delivery of services. Then, an additional need arises, and the cycle starts again. In the course of this process, reimbursement, employment opportunities, practice settings, and documentation change.

## Reimbursement

As resources become more limited, they become restricted to situations and conditions where they are most needed. Reimbursement has also become limited as PPS has come more to the forefront. Regulation of costs became necessary due to advancing medical costs, and the manner in which controls were implemented led to a reduction in services, which, in some cases, has led to ethical debate as to whether high-quality care is being delivered. The challenge of the health care system is to operate on a sound fiscal basis while providing care of high standards.

## Employment Opportunities

As funding shifts due to changes in legislation and financial resources change, so do employment opportunities. Following the advent of DRGs, long-term care facilities became a highly desirable place of employment for occupational therapy personnel, due to the increase in job availability following limitations in the acute setting. Opportunities were plentiful and salaries were good. Then, with the passage of the BBA, this scenario changed drastically. As noted in the history, OTs are now forging into new practice territory. In addition, as the market adjusts to changes imposed by legislation, the job market tends to stabilize.

## Practice Settings

As we have seen, occupational therapists find themselves applying their skills in different settings as markets shift. As a profession, OT has the advantage of having human occupation and performance as its focus. This allows us to focus on human performance in a variety of settings, opening wide doors of opportunity. We must be cognizant to apply ourselves based on premises of the profession and practice within our professional philosophies and parameters, and although all settings might not be the most appropriate for us, OTs have a great advantage in responding to needs in a variety of settings. This has never been more exemplified as the current movement toward new community settings.

## Documentation

As illustrated in the history, legislation and resultant changes impact the manner in which we report our services. As settings change, documentation content needs change, and as resources become more limited, third-party payers (in many cases the government) want to know exactly what they are paying for. The result is guidelines for documentation that will change as economic, social, and political environments change. Therefore, the OT practitioner must maintain a constant awareness of documentation requirements and guidelines.

Again, Chapter 5 outlines the specific impact that legislation has had on health care funding and its impact on occupational therapy practice.

# Summary

While many students tend to shy away from the "dry" topic of history, it can reveal much when observed in a certain manner. Hopefully, this brief account of some of the major legislative changes affecting occupational therapy has illustrated the old proverbial saying about one door closing and another opening. When a change occurs, there can be a positive effect.

The challenge comes when we must creatively manage practice to uphold our ethics, standards, and philosophies. Rosee (2000) speaks to the need to reconcile the demands of reimbursement systems, increased government surveillance, and providing services that demonstrate our efficacy as care providers and revenue generators.

# References

American Occupational Therapy Association. (1999, August 19). Strategic plan update: OT in the year 2010. *OT Week, 13*(2) 2-3.

Baum, C. (1997, June). The managed care system: The educator's opportunity. *The Education Special Interest Quarterly, 7*, 1-3.

Jacobs, K. (1996). The evolution of the occupational therapy delivery system. In AOTA (Ed.), *The occupational therapy manager* (Rev. ed.). Bethesda, MD: AOTA.

Peloquin, S. M. (1998). The therapeutic relationship. In M. E. Neistadt & E. B. Crepeau (Eds.), *Willard and Spackman's occupational therapy* (9th ed., pp. 105-119). Philadelphia: Lippincott.

Robnett, R. H. (1999). The continuum of care. In W. C. Chop & R. H. Robnett (Eds.), *Gerontology for the health care professional* (pp. 227-255). Philadelphia: F. A. Davis.

Rosee, M. (2000). The therapist as a fiscal manager: Surviving the SNF PPS and beyond. *OT Practice, 5*(9), 21-26.

Stancliff, B. L. (1997). Emerging practice areas: Going where no OT has gone before.... *OT Practice, 2*(7) 16-32.

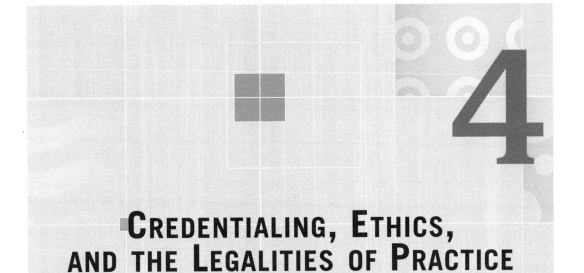

# Introduction

As health care professionals, occupational therapy practitioners must actively engage in responsible practice. This involves not only understanding and adhering to the ethics and legalities specific to occupational therapy (OT), but also health care policies in general. In this chapter, the occupational therapy assistant (OTA) will become familiar with the credentialing processes set forth by national organizations such as the American Occupational Therapy Association (AOTA), the National Board for Certification in Occupational Therapy (NBCOT), and the Accreditation Council for Occupational Therapy Education (ACOTE), as well as state licensure boards. Ethics and legal issues guiding the practice of occupational therapy will also be examined in this chapter.

## The Process of Credentialing

Credentialing is the process of qualifying an individual or organization based on "a predetermined set of standards such as licensure or certification—establishing that a person or institution has achieved professional recognition in a specific field of health care" (Rose, 1996, p. 603). There are two levels of credentialing within the scope of occupational therapy. For the registered occupational therapist (OTR), credential requires completing a 4-year baccalaureate or post-graduate program. As of 2007, the entry-level degree for the OTR credential is required to be at the master's level. The technical practitioner, the occupational therapy assistant, credential requires completing a 2-year associate's degree program. In addition to the academic requirements of either program, all occupational therapy practitioners are required to successfully complete supervised fieldwork and pass a national certification examination administered by the NBCOT. Occupational therapy standards are additionally independently regulated within each of the 50 states; Washington, DC; Guam; and Puerto Rico (AOTA, 2000a). Based on academic program accreditation and individual registration, occupational therapy was among the first health care professions to initiate a credentialing process. The process of registration (for OTRs) began in the form of a written essay examination. In 1947, the format was changed to a multiple choice answer examination, which remains to date. Although the 1950s saw the beginning of the practice of the occupational therapy assistant, it was not regulated via examination credentialing until 1977 (Gray, 1993).

Closely aligned with ethics and continuing competency, obtaining and maintaining current and appropriate certification and credentials sends a message to the public that occupational therapy "practitioners are trustworthy and accountable" (Opacich, 1996, p. 638). The credential processes set forth by NBCOT and state regulatory boards are designed to maintain the high standards associated with the practice of occupational therapy.

Currently, credentialing issues that appear to be impacting the profession include regulation of foreign-trained therapists and practice acts. Let's begin by looking at issues regarding foreign-trained therapists. It is imperative that foreign-trained, certified occupational therapists initiate the process of certification in the United States by first contacting NBCOT to determine specific requirement statutes, which include sitting for and successfully completing the certification examination (Rose, 1996).

For those students and practicing occupational therapists trained in Canada and Mexico, the North American Free Trade Agreement (NAFTA) permits (after receiving the necessary visa and immigration status) practice in the United States. It must be made clear that all therapists trained in Mexico or Canada are required to meet the same NBCOT requirements as domestically trained therapists (certification examination and state regulatory statutes) in order to work as an occupational therapy practitioner in the United States. It is through the practice provisions of the NAFTA treaty that new opportunities for occupational therapists trained in Mexico and Canada have arisen, which in turn has increased the pool of occupational therapy practitioners in the United States (Gray, 1993).

## Credentialing for Practitioners

Gray (1993) defines two types of credentialing that apply to individual practitioners:

### CERTIFICATION

This is a credential awarded to an individual who has successfully met a predetermined set of qualifications. It is a public recognition that designates an individual who has met certain standards and can only be used by those who have met the specified criteria. As defined in the State Regulation and Specialty Certification of Practitioners chapter of *The Occupational Therapy Manager,* certification is "the process by which an agency grants a person permission to use a certain title if that person has attained entry level competence; may be voluntary or mandatory as determined by state law; may also be governmental" (Rose, 1996, p. 603).

### STATE PRACTICE ACTS

State practice acts include legislation that is passed by individual states and that governs practice in a given discipline within that state. In order to practice legally, an occupational therapy practitioner must meet the criteria defined by the state practice act.

Table 4-1

### State Regulatory Practices

| LICENSURE | MANDATORY OR VOLUNTARY CERTIFICATION | REGISTRATION | TITLE CONTROL |
|---|---|---|---|
| 40 states, Guam, Puerto Rico, and District of Columbia | Indiana, Missouri, Vermont, Virginia, Wisconsin | Kansas, Michigan, Minnesota | Colorado, Hawaii |

Despite the fact that there is evidence suggesting that state regulation of various professions has existed since the 17th century, it was not until the 1970s that Florida and New York became the first states to regulate the practice of occupational therapy. Today, practice is regulated on a state by state basis. Therefore, each state is responsible for the implementation of specific laws and regulations governing the practice of occupational therapy (Rose, 1996).

State practice acts may take the following forms:

- *Licensure:* A process regulated by the government that grants permission for an individual to engage in certain professional practices. A practitioner must demonstrate a specified level of competency to be granted a license. Licensure is viewed as a practice that is in place to protect the public from unqualified practitioners.
- *Registration:* The practice of listing individuals on a roster maintained by government or private agencies. There may or may not be criteria or standards for being included on the roster. Registration may be voluntary or mandatory.
- *Title Control or Trademark:* Title control or trademark restricts the use of a particular title to an individual who has met specified certification requirements. In other words, if an individual has not completed the appropriate requirements, he or she may not call him- or herself an occupational therapy practitioner.

Table 4-1 provides a description of the types of regulatory processes imposed by each of the 50 states, the District of Columbia, Guam, and Puerto Rico.

## Credentialing for Programs and Organizations

Accreditation is the method by which a program or organization receives credentialing and which involves development, promotion, and ongoing re-evaluation of standards of excellence in occupational therapy education (NSPOT, 1917). Accreditation is awarded to a program that demonstrates it has met or exceeded a predetermined set of criteria (Gray, 1993). Accreditation may be granted to educational programs, health care organizations, schools, and other organizations.

The governing board overseeing this process is the Accreditation Council for Occupational Therapy Education (ACOTE). The mission statement of ACOTE includes four goals and objectives:

## FOSTER THE DEVELOPMENT AND ACCREDITATION OF QUALITY EDUCATIONAL PROGRAMS

- Set appropriately rigorous standards for occupational therapy/occupational therapy assistant education
- Accredit those programs which meet those standards
- Encourage the enhancement of educational programs
- Foster and reinforce importance of purposeful occupation

## IDENTIFY AND PROMOTE THE ONGOING DEVELOPMENT OF INDIVIDUALS WHO CAN PROVIDE LEADERSHIP FOR ACOTE NOW AND IN THE FUTURE

- Define and refine selection criteria for members of ACOTE and the Roster of Accreditation Evaluators (RAE)
- Develop an effective ACOTE/RAE application and screening process
- Recruit, educate, and retain ACOTE and RAE members
- Involve program directors, faculty, and others interested in educational opportunities designed for ACOTE/RAE members

## DEVELOP AND REFINE A COMPREHENSIVE ACOTE EVALUATION SYSTEM

- Examine current processes and procedures for effectiveness and efficacy
- Examine accreditation standards and processes for both content and outcomes
- Establish and implement valid and reliable outcome measures
- Propose changes in accreditation standards, processes, and procedures based on evaluation results

## APPLY TECHNOLOGY TO MAXIMIZE ACOTE FUNCTIONS

- Determine the technological needs of ACOTE and its communities of interest
- Prepare and implement a plan for acquiring state-of-the-art technology and educating ACOTE, RAE, ACES, etc. in its use
- Develop, implement, and maintain ACOTE website information related to ACOTE activities (AOTA, 1999a)

Within the profession of occupational therapy, and through rigorous principles such as those set forth by ACOTE, academic programs are upheld to the highest standards of moral and ethical practices (AOTA, 1999a). The AOTA has been responsible for the accreditation of occupational therapy education programs since 1935 (1999a). Today, there are more than 300 accredited occupational therapy programs in the United States, Washington DC, and Puerto Rico. Occupational therapy academic accreditation is described in the *Standards for an Accredited Educational Program for the Occupational Therapy Assistant*. The *Standards* provide the "minimum standards of quality used in establishing an accreditation of a program" (AOTA, 1998).

The *Standards* includes three sections:

- Section One: General Requirements for Accreditation—including sponsorship resources, students, operational policies, and program elevation
- Section Two: Specific Requirements for Accreditation—including curriculum content requirements and program length

- Section Three: Maintaining and Administering Accreditation—including program and sponsoring institution responsibilities and accreditation committee responsibilities.

For specific information regarding the guidelines for these essentials, the reader is directed to *Standards for an Accredited Educational Program for the Occupational Therapy Assistant*.

Excluding Colorado, Rhode Island, and Virginia, all states, as well as Puerto Rico, Guam, and the District of Columbia, regulate the practice of occupational therapy assistants (Rose, 1996). Table 4–2 indicates resources for information on practice regulation that each state (and US territory) imposes on its credentialed therapists.

The reader is directed to Table 4–3 for a timeline of credentialing milestones in the history of occupational therapy.

## Breaches of Certification

What transpires in the case of breach of certification? In this section, we will explore three infringements—negligence, malpractice, and fraud—and the consequences for such actions within the practice scope of the occupational therapy assistant.

Negligence refers to a "departure from the standard of due care toward others," including both deliberate and careless instances of enjoined risk to a patient or client. Negligence generally results when something is not done or neglected, resulting in an accident or mishap. Had neglect not occurred, the accident or mishap would likely have been avoided. According to Beauchamp and Childress, negligence indicates a "failure to meet moral obligations, including the failure to guard against risks of harm to others." For health care professionals, failure to provide a patient with "due care (to care or act reasonably toward others)" is considered an act of negligence. Although the standards for due care vary from setting to setting, as occupational therapy practitioners we are morally obligated to avoid engagement in negligent acts of any sort (Beauchamp & Childress, 1994, pp. 125-126).

Malpractice is actually a form of negligence. It occurs when a professional is found to have not followed an established "standard of care… [including] proper training, skills, and diligence." In order to be determined responsible for malpractice, the therapist must first be found negligent in acts of due care, and only then can it be established that the therapist did not meet "professional standards of care." If a practitioner engages in practice that they know they are not trained in, or if they engage in faulty judgment and decision-making and harm results to a recipient of care, malpractice may be said to have occurred (Beauchamp & Childress, 1994, p. 126).

As defined in *Black's Law Dictionary*, (1990, p. 660) fraud refers to "an intentional perversion of truth for the purpose of inducing another in reliance upon it to part with some valuable thing belonging to him or to surrender a legal right." Specific examples of fraud include falsification of client records, incorrect documentation, and payment fee alteration. Committing fraud is a direct breach of the Occupational Therapy Code of Ethics, and to be found blameworthy in matters of fraud, an occupational therapy practitioner is at risk for liability such as suspension or revocation of his or her state licensure to practice.

Now that we have reviewed the processes of credentialing, what comprises certification, and the impact of breaches of certification, let's explore the methods in which the certification process is monitored and enforced.

Table 4-2

## *Information Resources for State Credentialing*

| RESOURCE | DESCRIPTION OF INFORMATION |
|---|---|
| NBCOT www.nbcot.org | • From home page, link to "State Regulations." Provides explanation of state regulations and its implications.<br>• From home page, link to "Services." Provides verification of a practitioner's credentials. |
| AOTA www.aota.org | • Link to "Licensure" from home page. Log on at membership log-in page. Select from links to:<br>1. General information regarding state regulation and its importance.<br>2. Descriptions, by individual state, of practice laws, licensure fees, and continuing education requirements.<br>3. Contact information for the regulatory agencies of individual states. |

Table 4-3

## *Milestones in the OT Credentialing Process*

| | |
|---|---|
| 1923 | Minimum standards of training for occupational therapists established. |
| 1932 | First directory of qualified occupational therapists published, containing the names of 318 OTRs. A main register and secondary register, for persons qualified through work experience, are used. |
| 1937 | Registration requirements are changed. Only graduates of accredited schools are admitted to the registry. |
| 1939 | An essay examination is used for the registry. |
| 1947 | The first multiple-choice registration examination is administered. |
| 1957 | Plans approved for development of OTA training programs and certification as COTAs. |
| 1961 | First directory of COTAs published. There are 553 COTAs and six approved training programs. Some COTAs qualify under a grandfather program on the basis of work experience. |
| 1963 | Grandfather program for COTAs is discontinued. Certification requires graduation from an approved training program. |
| 1968 | Puerto Rico passes first licensure law for occupational therapists. |
| 1971 | AOTA Delegate Assembly passes resolution #300, the Continuing Certification Program. AOTA embarks on study of possible recertification policies and procedures. |

continued

Table 4-3 continued

## *Milestones in the OT Credentialing Process*

| | |
|---|---|
| 1971 | First COTA passes the certification examination for OTRs under the auspices of the Career Mobility Program. |
| 1973 | AOTA completes the Role Delineation Study for entry-level OTRs and COTAs. |
| 1975 | New York and Florida are first states to pass licensure laws for OTRs and COTAs. |
| 1977 | First certification exam for COTAs is administered. Certification as a COTA requires a passage of the certification examination. |
| 1982 | Career mobility program is terminated. |
| 1986 | AOTA membership approves by-laws change to create the American Occupational Therapy Certification Board (AOTCB) as a separate and autonomous entity under the auspices of the AOTA. |
| 1988 | AOTA membership approves by-laws change to allow for the creation of the AOTCB as a separate corporation, no longer affiliated with the AOTA. |
| 1990 | AOTCB publishes first issue of the *Disciplinary Action Information Exchange Network*. |
| 1991 | AOTCB Job Analysis Study completed. Results to be used to update certification exams to reflect current entry-level practice of OTRs and COTAs. |
| 1993 | A record-breaking number, over 5000, of candidates expected to take the certification exams. Effective with the January exams, the certification exams are changed to reflect changes in entry-level practice identified through the Job Analysis Study. |
| 1993 | A total of 30 jurisdictions have some form of regulation governing occupational therapists and occupational therapy assistants. |
| 1995 | The National Board for Certification in Occupational Therapy (NBCOT) assumes responsibilities for OT practitioner certification. |
| 2001 | NBCOT establishes requirements for continued professional competency for OT practitioners. |

Adapted from Ryan, S. (1995). *The combined volume: COTA* (2nd ed.) *and Practice issues in occupational therapy* (p. 313). Thorofare, NJ: SLACK Incorporated.

## *Enforcement Policies and Credentialing Agencies*

The agencies responsible for overseeing and enforcing matters involving credentialing include the NBCOT, ACOTE, and state boards. Although AOTA is considered our national professional organization, it is not a credentialing agency per se, as membership is voluntary. However, the AOTA established the standards for practice that have been adopted by most states (AOTA, 2000b). It is important to note that the Standards and Ethics Commission (SEC) is one of three commissions within the AOTA. All members of AOTA, including OTRs, COTAs, students, and associates fall within the jurisdiction of the SEC. Any type of disciplinary action and subsequent enforcement procedures fall within the scope of the Occupational Therapy Code of Ethics set forth by the SEC. The procedures defined in the scope of the Code are designed to permit AOTA to act in a fair manner in upholding the standards of the profession, while also safeguarding the rights of members against whom a complaint has been issued (AOTA, 1996). The principles of the SEC are designed to identify, inform, and educate members of AOTA about current trends in ethical issues; uphold practice and education standards; and to review all allegations of unethical conduct. Many of the complaints heard by the SEC are similar to those brought to either the NBCOT or to state regulatory boards. They include issues of sexual misconduct, fraudulent documentation, non-adherence to contracts, and professional incompetence in issues of provision of direct services. Above and beyond the aforementioned, complaints unique only to the SEC concern ethical issues such as plagiarism, supervision of students or staff, misrepresentation of research findings, and incompetence in teaching (www.promoteot.org, 1996). Although the SEC sets forth disciplinary actions independent of that of the NBCOT or state regulatory boards, the SEC routinely notifies NBCOT of complaints that have been received. As a protective measure against those involved in a disciplinary case, the SEC will often delay its disciplinary actions until NBCOT acts on the case.

Certification of practitioners was originally a duty and function of the AOTA. NBCOT was created in the 1980s in response to concerns over potential conflict of interest between AOTA's desire to promote further growth of the profession while also serving to protect the public against "unqualified professionals" (Rose, 1996). Consequently, the NBCOT functions independently of AOTA and serves as the national organization responsible for the initial certification of occupational therapy practitioners (Kyler, 2000). It also functions separately from state regulatory boards. However, many states regulating occupational therapy mandate that in order for a practitioner to be eligible for state certification, he or she hold initial NBCOT certification (Rose, 1996) and graduate from an accredited school, in addition to other individual (state) requirements.

The goals of NBCOT are to " promote public health, safety, and welfare by establishing, maintaining, and administering standards, policies, and programs" of its occupational therapy practitioners. To achieve certification by NBCOT, the practitioner must complete all educational, fieldwork, and examination requirements. Although the national board examinations for OTR and OTA contain differing content materials, both are comprised of 200 multiple-choice questions designed to measure entry-level competence on the part of the practitioner (1996, p. 613).

# Ethics

It is important to grasp the fundamental nature of credentialing, as it provides a solid foundation to build upon and understand the nature of ethical and legal practice. In addition to adhering to the ethical standards of practice set forth by the SEC, ACOTE, state regulatory boards, and NBCOT, as health care professionals, we are also guided by general biomedical ethical standards. Biomedical ethics takes into account "obtaining relevant information and assessing its reliability, identifying moral problems, and mapping out alternative solutions to the problems that have been previously identified." When we develop personal, moral, and ethical standards, it is only then that we are able to analyze and defend our actions and claims and function in a professional manner befitting the standards of the profession of occupational therapy (Beauchamp & Childress, 1994, p. 21).

Ethics are defined as the "careful and systematic study of morality. [Morality is then considered to be] a set of guidelines and standards that are striven for as ideals, to protect basic human values" (Bailey & Schwartzberg, 1995, p. 2). The study of ethics concerns such issues as "right versus wrong, justice, equality, free will, and responsibility" (Bloom, 1994, p. 52). According to Cummings (1993, pp. 299-300), ethics encompass "rightness or wrongness of an action." Ethical principles are based upon four standards: prudence, choosing the right means; temperateness, moderation; courage, being willing to do what is known as right; and justice, treating people "with integrity and honor."

Ethical behaviors guiding the practice of occupational therapy include: universalism, remaining non-biased in the manner in which we treat all patients; disinterestedness, not being motivated solely by money and always providing the best possible patient care (does not mean forsaking payment); and cooperation, working in a collegial manner and willingness to share knowledge (Cummings, 1993).

Ethical theories may be considered as two-fold: teleological—focusing on the consequences of an action, and deontologic—actions are right in and of themselves (one is duty-bound to do the right thing) (1993). Exploring what constitutes a "moral life" describes ethics from a "normative or descriptive" perspective. Normative ethics asks the question, "which action guides are worthy of moral acceptance and for what reasons... [while] descriptive ethics is the factual investigation of moral behavior and beliefs." Differentiating between the two types of ethics involves an understanding that descriptive ethics do not attempt to provide a "prescriptive guideline" (Beauchamp & Childress, 1994, pp. 9-10), while a normative ethical stance evokes an action-oriented position. The processes of defining an ethical code of standards are based on moral principles and standards, which include autonomy, beneficence, nonmaleficence, justice, (and others that govern) relationships (Opacich, 1996).

Autonomy is defined as the "condition of being self governing" (Morris, 1981, p. 90). The Code of Ethics collectively encompasses qualities involving autonomy, privacy, and confidentiality such that the "occupational therapy practitioners shall collaborate with service recipients or their surrogate(s) in setting goals and priorities throughout the intervention process" (AOTA, 2000a, p. 2). In the realm of occupational therapy, autonomy, or self-determination, adjuncts that individuals have the right and ability to know what is in their best interest. To help guide patients in this process of self-determination, therapists must provide viable options from which patients may make informed decisions. Facilitating and providing patients with a sense of autonomy necessitates respect for patient dignity in all facets of care. Today, practitioners are being called upon to participate in team meetings and discussions directly involving patient autonomy. Meeting these challenges as occupational therapy practitioners and managers involves providing the most ethical level of patient care and becoming well versed in protocols and legislative issues relating to issues of autonomy (Opacich, 1996). One of the ways autonomy is preserved is by obtaining informed consent from patients. Informed consent is an agreement, signed by a patient or their representative, which states that treatment is agreed upon after a thorough explanation of procedures and their risks and benefits. Patients reserve the right to refuse treatment as part of their autonomy. It is also the practitioner's responsibility to exercise beneficence, and advise the patient regarding the consequences of refusing treatment. The ultimate decision, however, remains with the patient.

Beneficence, as described by Opacich, encompasses "actions that benefit others, including, but not limited to acts of mercy, kindness, and charity" (1996, p. 632). In Principle One of the Code of Ethics, beneficence is defined as "occupational therapy personnel shall demonstrate a concern for the well-being of the recipients of their services" (AOTA, 2000a, p. 1). It implies that an individual must actively engage in acts considered to be good, while also concurrently considering any potential for harm in patient care. When acting in a beneficent manner, a therapist must weigh the tendency to act in a manner known as paternalism (the presumption that by virtue of experience, the health care provider knows what is best in terms of patient care) with the right for a patient to make active choices in medical care options (Opacich, 1996, p. 632). In its application to the practice of occupational therapy, beneficence refers to the practitioner's "duty to act for the patient's good" (Bailey & Schwartzberg, 1995, p. 4). To better assist the patient in making informed choices, and thereby strengthening the moral standard of beneficence in patient care, it is the responsibility of the occupational therapy practitioner to become well versed in efficacy and benefit outcomes studies. Knowing research results and understanding the implications of evidence-based practice are part of ethical practice. The significance of understanding research and outcome studies will be addressed in Chapter 9.

Nonmaleficence refers to the ideal of the "Hippocratic tradition of doing no harm" (Opacich, 1996, p. 632). Principle Two of the Code of Ethics defines nonmaleficence as "precautions to avoid imposing or inflicting harm upon the recipient of services or to his or her property" (AOTA, 2000b, p. 2). It refers to acting in a diligent and responsible manner at all times, or in legal terms to provide what is known as "due care" (Bailey & Schwartzberg, 1995, p. 5). Simply stated, as occupational therapy practitioners, we must at all times avoid inflicting harm of any type upon our patients. Issues of nonmaleficence have frequently been debated in occupational therapy in terms of quality of life, withdrawal of treatment, passive and active euthanasia, etc. (Opacich, 1996). It is very important to maintain an ongoing self-dialogue regarding issues of nonmaleficence. As an occupational therapy practitioner, staying abreast of current ethical issues is of great assistance in formulating personal ethical standards.

In terms of the occupational therapy practitioner, Principle Five of the Code ("Justice") states that "occupational therapy personnel shall comply with laws and Association policies guiding the profession of occupational therapy" (AOTA, 2000a, p. 3). According to Bailey and Schwartzberg (1995, p. 7), justice contains two components: noncomparative and comparative. Comparative justice refers to a patient receiving something that he or she is entitled to receive. The branch of comparative justice that most significantly impacts the health care professions is called *distributive justice*. It asks questions such as "is everyone entitled to receive health care benefits, and if so, is everyone entitled to the same amount?" When dealing with such a dilemma, the therapist may decide that treating similar "cases in similar ways" may be the just and fair way to carry out therapy services. Noncomparative justice attends to the "application of laws and rules to the distribution of burdens and benefits." Prioritization of services in a moral and just manner is one of the most challenging functions of the occupational therapy manager, especially in the current era of limited funding and resources.

Utility fits best with beneficence and nonmaleficence in that it guides in establishing order when there are "competing needs" such as "who will be treated, treatment methods, and frequency of treatment" (Bailey & Schwartzberg, 1995, p. 6). These questions and moral standards often result in varying degrees of ethical dilemma. The Code of Ethics also describes principles of duty, veracity, and fidelity (AOTA, 2000b). Collectively, these seven principles comprise the ethical standards from which our profession is to be implemented.

While considered to be aspirational, rather than legal, in nature, all practitioners at every level of practice must be aware of and fully understand the Guidelines to the Occupational

Therapy Code of Ethics, the Code of Ethics, and Core Values and Attitudes of Occupational Therapy Practice. As set forth by the AOTA, these collective documents "serve as moral and philosophical statements that encourage occupational therapy practitioners to attain a high level of professional behavior... [and] bind the profession to the singular purpose of assuring the public of high quality occupational therapy services" (Hansen, 1998, p. 881).

The Guidelines to the Occupational Therapy Code of Ethics provides the practitioner with information regarding morally correct practice standards and behaviors and provides direction to the OT practitioner in interpreting and applying the Code of Ethics. It also serves as a guide in clarifying complex moral and ethical questions (Hansen, 1998). The Occupational Therapy Code of Ethics was recently revised, setting forth seven principles to "promote and maintain high standards of behavior in occupational therapy" (AOTA, 2000). The topics covered in the Guidelines to the Occupational Therapy Code of Ethics include honesty, communication, ensuring the common good, competence, confidentiality, conflict of interest, the impaired practitioner, sexual relationships, and payment for services.

As previously discussed, the Occupational Therapy Code of Ethics applies to occupational therapy personnel at all levels of practice. Any violations of the code are considered to be unethical acts and are enforced by the SEC. Enforcement of the Occupational Therapy Code of Ethics is carried out in a thorough and systematic manner. As mandated by the SEC, "any action that is in violation of the spirit and purpose of this Code shall be considered unethical" (AOTA, 2000a). Further, and perhaps considered an intrinsic quality of the profession, occupational therapy practitioners are obligated to maintain a high standard of professional ethics and to "promote and support" them among colleagues. Should an action be deemed as a violation of the Code, the SEC of the AOTA may take disciplinary procedures, which may take the following forms:

- *Reprimand:* Formal expression of disapproval of conduct communicated privately by letter from the chairperson of the SEC
- *Censure:* A formal expression of disapproval that is public
- *Suspension*: Removal of membership for a specified period of time
- *Revocation:* Permanent denial of membership
- *Dismissal of charges* (AOTA, 2000a)

The SEC of the AOTA has authority over membership in AOTA. Actions executed by the SEC do not affect a practitioner's right to practice. Readers are urged to familiarize themselves with the document entitled Enforcement Procedure for Occupational Therapy Code of Ethics available at www.aota.org to gain further insight into the disciplinary procedures set forth by the SEC.

NBCOT has the authority to suspend or revoke a practitioner's COTA or OTR credential, therefore giving NBCOT the potential to remove one's right to practice. NBCOT may take any of the following actions in the event that a breach of ethics is determined:

- *Ineligibility for certification*: An individual is barred from becoming certified by the NBCOT, either indefinitely or for a certain duration.
- *Reprimand:* A formal expression of disapproval, which is retained in the certificant's file, but remains private.
- *Censure:* A formal expression of disapproval that is made public.
- *Probation:* Continued certification is subject to fulfillment of specified conditions (e.g., monitoring, education, supervision, and/or counseling).

- *Suspension:* The loss of certification for a specified amount of time. The individual may have to apply for reinstatement following the duration of the suspension.
- *Revocation:* Certification is permanently removed.

The NBCOT website (www.nbcot.org) provides additional detail regarding the purpose, grounds, and procedures for disciplinary action. NBCOT communicates disciplinary action with a practitioner's state licensing board and state associations (NBCOT, 2002).

State regulatory boards have jurisdiction over practitioners in their respective states and maintain the authority to invoke similar sanctions on a practitioner for violation of the state's practice act.

Core Values and Attitudes of Occupational Therapy Practice was developed by the SEC in an effort to define the "attitudes and values that undergird the profession of occupational therapy" (Kanny, 1993, p. 1085). The outcome of the study was a compilation of seven terms best describing the values and attitudes of occupational therapists, including altruism, equality, freedom, justice, dignity, truth, and prudence. While all of these terms are thought to inherently describe the practice of occupational therapy, the way in which they are incorporated into practice varies within different work environments. One of the most important ideals set forth by Core Values and Attitudes of Occupational Therapy Practice is the "challenge" to possess clear understanding of one's personal values and align them into the common framework of those of the profession of occupational therapy (Kanny, 1993).

## Ethical Reasoning

The process of ethical reasoning can be best defined in terms of its relationship to clinical reasoning. It is through use of ethical reasoning that occupational therapy practitioners base their decisions in the role of clinician, educator, researcher, or manager. When discussing ethical reasoning, it is often individual moral constructs that lead a practitioner to experience a sense of ambivalence when faced with a team-based therapy option or request that makes him or her uncomfortable. This feeling of unbalance and unrest contributes to what is known as ethical tension. Recognizing it to be a tension-provoking situation is the first step in the ethical reasoning process. From this point, it is the responsibility of the practitioner to become well-acquainted with ethical concepts and principles that best articulate his or her concerns. Finally, the practitioner/manager must develop a strategy designed to lead to a resolution of ethical conflict. By nature, occupational therapy practitioners are dedicated to honoring and validating patients, rights, and values (Opacich, 1996).

Please refer to Figure 4-1 for a visual schema of ethical reasoning as prepared by G. Bloom (1994).

Historically, ethics have played an important role in the occupational therapy management process by defining the entire scope of practice; the why, when, what if, and how occupational therapy is carried forth. Currently, several ethical issues in occupational therapy management are receiving a great deal of attention. These situations constitute what are known as ethical dilemmas, which "exists when no single satisfactory choice or answer is appropriate for a certain situation, or when there are only less-than-satisfactory alternatives" (Bailey & Schwartzberg, 1995, p. 2). They include managed care, limited resources, and diversity issues. In terms of managed care and with the sky rocketing costs of health care and delivery systems, as occupational therapy practitioners, we are faced with many moral and ethical dilemmas. The dilemma arises from what we internally know as the right course of care versus the external physical, and fiscal constraints placed upon us. Being called upon to most effectively deal with these ethical dilemmas is a reality in today's practice of occupational therapy. Additionally, accepting and learning from the diverse cultural and spiritual

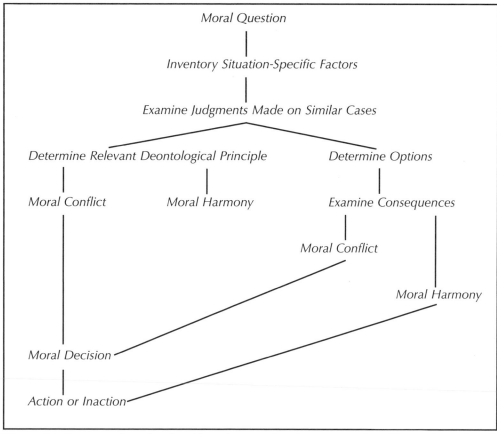

**Figure 4-1.** Steps to solve ethical problems (reprinted with permission from Bloom, G. M. [1994]. Ethical issues in occupational therapy. In K. Jacobs, & M. K. Logigian [Eds.], *Functions of a manager in occupational therapy* [Rev. ed., p. 59]. Thorofare, NJ: SLACK Incorporated).

backgrounds of colleagues and patients may initially present a challenge to practitioners, yet ultimately reinforce the holistic nature of the profession.

Engaging in dialogue with patients, families, and other health care professionals is an important part of ethical problem solving. In the role of occupational therapy assistant manager, the practitioner must be open minded in dealing with a myriad of ethical concerns. In particular, Opacich (1996, p. 637) defines four ethical duties that the (OT) manager must perform. They include, "(1) facilitation of ethical clinical decision making; (2) professional gatekeeping (ensuring the competence of practitioners); (3) allocation of limited resources; and (4) enhancement of the organization's and employees' integrity." As a profession, we formulate ethical directives in our practice as bound by the Occupational Therapy Code of Ethics. Not only must a manager actively assist in ethical decision making; he or she must also guide staff and colleagues in defining their scope of ethical insight. This is done through meaningful discussion and dialogue with others in what is known as a "diverse spectrum of cultures and beliefs" (p. 637) as well as through reading and self-reflection. The ultimate goal of ethical practice is the provision of the most competent and morally just level of patient care in all situations, at all times. It is the skilled and empathic manager who deals with these ethical issues in a professional manner and ultimately makes final decisions on the basis of "intellectual inquiry and not emotion" (Bloom, 1994).

# Law and Ethics in Practice

As health care practitioners, we are ethically, morally, and legally bound to practice service the best way possible. We must avoid at all times, any situations that compromise the Centers for Medicare and Medicaid Services (CMS) regulations (i.e., any type of Medicare/Medicaid fraud in billing, incorrect documentation, or any other issues that compromise not only oneself, but the profession of occupational therapy). Being a role model to colleagues and staff is the first step in sound ethical practice. Should you determine that an ethical or legal violation has potentially occurred within the scope of your practice, before making the decision to file any type of formal ethics-based complaint, it is important to consider these points:

1. What are your expectations regarding the outcome of your dilemma?
2. What answers can be derived from your state regulatory board? As each state sets forth different laws governing occupational therapy practice issues, starting on a more local level is the proactive stance to adopt.
3. Based on the work setting that you are practicing within, have you made yourself familiar with existing policies and procedures that impact your concerns? Further, have you consulted with your supervisor, or spoken in confidence with personnel from human resources or the employee assistance program at your job site?
4. Should you seek legal counsel?
5. After going through the aforementioned channels, what are your current expectations regarding the outcome of your concerns? (Kyler, 2000)

Situations may arise in which it may be advisable to seek legal counsel. Examples may include situations wherein your actions may conflict with the views or positions of your employer, situations where your actions on behalf of yourself or your employer may lead to potential liability to patients and/or their families, and situations wherein your actions, or inaction, may place you at risk of violation of laws or regulations of professional or local governing agencies. In all instances, care should be taken to determine the appropriate course of action for the situation.

At a minimum, proper documentation of the entire situation should be created and maintained. Keeping timely, complete, and accurate records of your actions and treatment can go a long way to helping support your position and provides an outsider (such as an attorney, or a judge or jury who is later introduced to the situation) with a clear view of the events involved. Such records should include a log or journal outlining dates and times of any happenings, meetings, or communications relating to the situation. All relevant facts should be delineated, including the details of the situation; any conversations or meetings relating to the situation; who the participants are; what their instructions, positions, or views are; and any written communications or reports relating to the situation. Wherever possible, attempt to get communications in writing or summarize oral communications in writing as soon as practicable.

If you feel that consultation with an attorney is warranted, it is important to determine the type of attorney necessary for the particular situation. If your situation involves liability for you and your employer, your employer may direct you to an attorney that represents your employer as well as yourself, since your interests may be similar. Such an attorney may have expertise in medical malpractice, insurance law, criminal law, health care law, Americans with Disabilities Act (ADA), Individuals with Disabilities Education Act (IDEA), or local health care regulations depending on the situation. Care, however, should be exercised in that to the extent your interests may conflict with your employer's, it would be advisable to seek an independent attorney to represent your interests first and foremost. For example, if you are concerned that your job or reputation as a practitioner may be at risk because your actions conflict with the positions of your employer, despite a strong feeling that your actions are correct professionally and/or ethically, seeking counsel from your own employment attorney might be appropriate.

If you decide to seek advice of an attorney, those with the appropriate experience may be found through inquiry with state and local bar associations. Like occupational therapy practitioners, attorneys must be licensed to practice through their respective state bars. Many state bars have web sites where information on licensed attorneys is available. Of course, recommendations from those who have had previous dealings with particular attorneys can be particularly helpful.

Typically, an initial consultation with an attorney is at a nominal flat fee or even free of charge. At this consultation, you can explain the facts surrounding your situation to the attorney and receive preliminary legal advice relating to your case as well as an outline of the potential options for proceeding forward. These consultations are considered confidential communications between you and your attorney, and are subject to both the attorney-client privilege and the attorney's ethical duty of confidentiality. The attorney-client privilege prevents a court from disclosing the confidential communications between an attorney and his or her client when that communication concerns the professional relationship between them. This privilege includes the aforementioned initial consultation, even if you ultimately do not hire that attorney to represent you. The ethical duty of confidentiality, a broader protection that applies in instances where the attorney-client privilege does not, prevents an attorney from disclosing or using any information relating to the representation of a client unless that client consents to such disclosure.

One final point regarding seeking legal advice is worth considering. Attorneys are under an ethical obligation to avoid representing clients where a conflict of interest may be present. When seeking an attorney to represent your interests, it would be prudent to ask in advance whether they are currently, or have previously, represented any potential adversaries (including the aforementioned patients, families, employers, etc.). If so, it may be advisable to seek another attorney without a similar conflict of interest, rather than relate the details of your situation to this attorney.

The decision to seek legal advice should be carried out with careful thought and full consideration of all the parties and issues involved. Depending on the specific situation, your interests as an occupational therapist may be aligned with, or opposed to, those of your patient, your employer, or other third-party. While a serious step, it is important for the comprehensive protection of your patients and your profession, as well as your personal interests, that you consider seeking appropriate advice of counsel upon the appearance of legal or ethical issues in your practice.

Ethical practice, credentialing, regulatory boards, and the creation of practice standards unite to achieve a common goal—the provision of high-quality occupational therapy services. Ethical guidelines set the ideals that all COTA practitioners should strive for in their practice. Ethical practice not only directly impacts the practitioner, but also the patient, his or her family, and society as a whole. Maintaining and upholding the standards set forth by AOTA, NBCOT, and state regulatory boards are also of critical importance to the COTA practitioner. Such regulatory and associated credentialing processes establish uniform minimal proficiency standards, and in doing so, ensure that all COTA practitioners are appropriately trained in a consistent manner. These standards and regulatory processes not only ensure a high quality of practice, but also ultimately protect the public and the credibility of the profession itself.

## Case study

Jason, a newly certified COTA, was just notified by NBCOT that he passed the certification examination. Jason was a diligent student, and in addition to maintaining a high grade-point average, worked as a nursing assistant in a skilled-care facility while attending school. Jason's schedule at the facility prevented him from spending more than a few moments here and there observing in the occupational therapy clinic, yet he felt confident that he had chosen the right career path. Jason was well liked by the nursing staff and administration and performed his role with responsibility and compassion. Based on the recommendation of the head nurse, he was asked to stay on after graduation in the role of a COTA, working under the direct supervision of an OTR with 5 years of experience. Despite the fact that Jason had an offer to remain on as a COTA at his Level II Fieldwork, a public school district, he felt a sense of personal honor and loyalty to continue working at the skilled nursing facility. After taking a brief vacation following the certification exam, Jason eagerly began his career as a COTA.

All was progressing smoothly for Jason at work. Over the first few months his supervisor began giving Jason more challenging tasks, such as leading small group and invited him to sit on the interdisciplinary professional counsel at the facility. Gradually, Jason began to notice that his supervisor was becoming increasingly unavailable not only to Jason, but to the patients. She did not appear to be granting patients the autonomy that Jason thought they deserved, and instead of inviting patients and families to actively participate in treatment planning, began to insist that she was the "expert," and as such, only her opinion was of any value. One day while Jason was preparing to write a note in a patient's chart, he noticed that his supervisor had written notes for treatment and subsequent third-party reimbursement that had not really taken place. In fact, the supervisor had not even been at work on several of these days.

After spending an agonizing night thinking about the situation, Jason decided that he would speak directly with his supervisor and discuss his concerns. His supervisor became very defensive and threatened to not only fire Jason, but ruin his future as a COTA if he voiced his concerns to anyone else. Jason was experiencing an ethical dilemma. Not only did he recognize evidence of potential fraud, he could have potentially lost his license and precipitated an investigation of the faculty. Ultimately, Jason decided to reapproach his supervisor and explain that morally and ethically he could not ignore this situation. He brought a copy of the AOTA's Occupational Therapy Code of Ethics to add support to his stance. After an angry exchange of words, Jason and the supervisor spoke with the director of the facility to discuss the ramifications of the supervisor's actions. Based on an investigation by the SEC, the supervisor's license to practice occupational therapy was suspended, and the nursing facility issued her a termination of employment notice. After this experience, Jason determined that he wanted to become even more versed in issues of ethics and subsequently became a leading expert on issues of health care-related ethics.

# References

American Occupational Therapy Association, Government Relations Department. (1996). *Scope of SEC disciplinary action program.* Bethesda, MD: Author.

American Occupational Therapy Association. (1998). *Standards for an accredited educational program for the occupational therapy assistant* (on-line). Retrieved November 4, 2002, from www.aota.org/nonmembers/area13/docs/otasf.doc

American Occupational Therapy Association, Government Relations Department. (1999a). *Accreditation council for occupational therapy education.* Retrieved September 5, 2002, from http://www.aota.org/nonmembers/area13/links/LINK20.asp

American Occupational Therapy Association, Government Relations Department. (1999b). About us. Bethesda, MD: Author.

American Occupational Therapy Association, Government Relations Department. (2000a). *Occupational therapy code of ethics.* Bethesda, MD: Author.

American Occupational Therapy Association. (2000b) *Enforcement procedures for occupational therapy code of ethics.* Retrieved September 11, 2002 from, http://www.aota.org/members/area2/links/link07.asp

Anderson, K. N. (1994). *Mosby's medical, nursing, and allied heath dictionary* (4th ed). St. Louis, MO: Mosby.

Bailey, D. M., & Schwartzberg, S. L. (1995). *Ethical and legal dilemmas in occupational therapy.* Philadelphia: F.A. Davis.

Beauchamp, T. L., & Childress, J. F. (1994). *Principles of biomedical ethics.* New York: Oxford University Press.

Black, H. C. (1990). *Black's law dictionary* (6th ed.). St. Paul, MN: West Publishing Co.

Bloom, G. M. (1994). Ethical issues in occupational therapy. In K. Jacobs, & M. K. Logigian (Eds.), *Functions of a manager in occupational therapy* (Rev. ed., pp. 52-66). Thorofare, NJ: SLACK Incorporated.

Cummings, G., Sr. (1993). Principles of occupational therapy ethics. In S. E. Ryan (Ed.), *Practice issues in occupational therapy: Intraprofessional team building* (pp. 299-307). Thorofare, NJ: SLACK Incorporated.

Gray, M. (1993). The credentialing process in occupational therapy. In S. E. Ryan (Ed.), *Practice issues in occupational therapy: Intraprofessional team building* (pp. 307-314). Thorofare, NJ: SLACK Incorporated.

Hansen, R.A. (1998). Guidelines to the occupational therapy code of ethics. *Am J Occup Ther, 52*(10), 881-884.

Kanny, E. (1993). Core values and attitudes of occupational therapy practice. *Am J Occup Ther, 47*(12), 1085-1086.

Kyler, P. (2000). *Frequently asked questions about ethics.* Retrieved September 5, 2002, from http://www.aota.org/members/area2/links/link17.asp

Morris, W. (Ed.). (1981). *The American heritage dictionary of the English language.* Boston: Houghton Mifflin.

National Society for the Promotion of Occupational Therapy. (1917). *Articles of incorporation.* Author.

Opacich, K. J. (1996). Ethical dimensions in occupational therapy. In J. B. Cox, J. Luschin, J. Brady, P. Kyler-Hutchinson, B. G. Manoly, S. Hertfelder, et al. (Eds.), *The occupational therapy manager* (pp. 627-650). Bethesda, MD: AOTA.

Rose, B. W. (1996). State regulation and specialty certification of practitioners. In J. B. Cox, J. Luschin, J. Brady, P. Kyler-Hutchinson, B. G. Manoly, S. Hertfelder, et al. (Eds.), *The occupational therapy manager* (pp. 603-625). Bethesda, MD: AOTA.

Ryan, S. (1995). *The combined volume: COTA* (2nd ed.) *and Practice issues in occupational therapy* (p. 313). Thorofare, NJ: SLACK Incorporated.

# Bibliography

National Board for Certification in Occupational Therapy. (2002). *Procedures for disciplinary action.* Retrieved September 5, 2002, from http://www.nbcot.org/nbcot/scripts/programs/disciplinary_action_procedures.asp

Quiroga, V. A. M. (1995). *Occupational therapy: The first thirty years, 1900-1930.* Bethesda, MD: AOTA.

# 5

# REIMBURSEMENT AND FINANCE

*Pamela DiPasquale-Lehnerz, MS, OTR*

## Introduction

For obvious reasons, *reimbursement*, or payment for services, is critical to all practice settings and facilities. Because reimbursement is controlled by corporate and regulatory factors, it is essential that occupational therapy personnel be familiar with both business and legal issues. The purpose of this chapter is to acquaint the student with types of reimbursement plans, the laws that affect reimbursement for occupational therapy (OT) services, and business concepts that contribute to a financially sound practice. The relationship between legislation, reimbursement, and trends in the profession will be elucidated. So that the student will understand the relationship of documentation and clinical decision-making to the reimbursement process, the reimbursement review process will be examined.

The student is also asked to bear in mind the relationship of reimbursement standards and legislation to opportunities to practice leadership and innovation in occupational therapy. As laws and regulatory agencies exert their influence, new markets that benefit from OT services become apparent. For example, the reduction of Medicare Part A (inpatient) coverage and the implementation of Medicare Part B that provides coverage for outpatient services limited reimbursement for inpatient services. Occupational therapists, although more limited in inpatient settings, found a new niche in outpatient services. This type of evolution continues today in different ways.

The student is reminded that the laws governing health care are constantly in flux and change quickly. Refer to Chapter 3 for a review of the history of the changes in health care legislation. Reimbursement is closely related to legislation. The information presented in this chapter is accurate and relevant as of this writing. By the time the finished piece finds its way to your OT management class, some of what is described in this chapter may be modified in one way or another, thereby affecting practice in different ways. The student is reminded that it is the practitioner's responsibility to know the regulations that are pertinent to their area of practice and to maintain current information regarding reimbursement issues. Use this information to understand the reimbursement process and the concerns that influence it, but be informed of and prepared for ongoing changes.

# Skills You Will Apply

## Management Skills

Many of the financial considerations of an occupational therapy department come under the heading of management skills, as they encompass budgeting, staffing, and productivity issues. Attending to revenue, costs, and the "bottom line" are closely related to management tasks. The COTA contributes to this by monitoring patient care, use of supplies, and by managing time wisely.

## Credentialing and Regulatory Standards

Reimbursement by Medicare and other third party payers is regulated by both federal and state laws. In turn, the facility's accreditation and license to operate are affected by compliance with regulations regarding reimbursement. Additionally, the practitioner is responsible, legally and ethically, to comply with reimbursement requirements. The relationship of finance to credentialing and regulatory guidelines is clear.

## Quality Assurance

Because financial considerations are a large part of the overall functioning and credibility of a department, they directly relate to the quality of the department.

# Overview of Regulation and Occupational Therapy Services

Reimbursement of occupational therapy services has been influenced by social, political, and economic climates from the origin of reconstruction aides of World War I, through the Great Depression, World War II, the economic boom of the '50s, the recession of the '70s, and up to the expansion of rehabilitation of the '90s. In all of these situations, political climate and regulatory demands have required that occupational therapists respond by altering the provision of services and meeting the demand for new services. Occupational therapists have expanded the types of services provided from psychiatry, vocational technical services in consolation houses, to reconstruction services to the war wounded in hospitals, to tuberculosis and polio patients, and to community-based mental health and public school systems. In each of these cases, occupational therapists have met the challenge to provide services in accordance with changing policies and reimbursement standards. In doing so, they have moved to new practice arenas and contributed to the growth and evolution of the profession. The challenge to provide those services by proper adherence to national standards, accreditation, medical documentation, and coding and outcome tracking has been met and continues to be modified.

The influence of standards and regulation dates back to the beginning of our history as a recognized profession. The groundwork for reimbursement was solidified by the 1920s, with the establishment of national standards for academic preparation and training. At the 1921 annual meeting of the National Society of the Promotion of Occupational Therapy, Eleanor Clarke Slagle addressed the membership on the procurement of a physicians order, stating that a prescription is necessary for the protection of the patient and OT practititoner (Quiroga, 1995). In the 1920s, communication between AOTA and other medical groups was enhanced (1995). As the profession sought recognition in the medical world, it was necessary to meet standards and to comply with established organizations that controlled the service delivery environment at the time. This set the stage for compliance with regulations and standards that affected reimbursement for professional services.

With occupational therapy firmly established in the medical model, the profession realized its future depended on the health care trends. A reimbursable service, separate from other rehabilitation services, became apparent to serve returning World War II veterans. By the 1970s, the provision of services spanned the service delivery settings from acute care to outpatient, home health, skilled nursing facilities, and long-term care options. The government mandated prospective payment system for diagnostic-related groups (DRGs) in the '80s, thus limiting the reimbursement to hospitals for acute care. This may have been a prime factor in the expansion of post acute services including the above and the emergence of transitional or subacute services. Because DRGs affected only the inpatient setting, services moved to outpatient settings and spurred the growth of community-based intervention.

The escalation in health care expenditures, especially for Medicare's post-acute care benefits, developed into a health care policy concern and led to health care reform initiatives. This was due to an increase in costs from about $2.5 billion in 1986 to more than $30 billion in 1996. Policy makers became concerned that utilization of Medicare benefits had become excessive and was not supporting any improvements in health or care (Liu et al., 1999). This contributed to the passage of the 1997 Balance Budget Act (BBA), which dramatically affected the provision of occupational therapy.

Survival of OT in the last part of the 20th century became dependent on successful negotiation in a complex health care system influenced by the need to meet standards and requirements of varying reimbursement sources. Both public and private funding sources increased in variation under the influence of managed care. Occupational therapists had to meet the challenges of network systems of care, which rose from large health care systems and health maintenance organization (HMO) requirements. Occupational therapy reimbursement was now, in part, dependent upon the level of documentation provided by the medical record and proper coding for reimbursement. Successful reimbursement depended upon understanding various network or contract requirements and incorporating them into daily practice. Reimbursement depends on the practitioner's knowledge and understanding of the various systems and requirements of their facility and the patient or client group they serve.

The following sections of this chapter will explain the various methods of reimbursement that have developed over the years, and the legislation and sociopolitical climates in which they evolved. Each of these provided the OT field with an opportunity for growth.

# Types of Reimbursement and Payment Systems

In order to build and understanding of the terminology used in this section, see Table 5–1, which defines terms that will be used in the explanation of reimbursement systems.

## Fee for Service

This type of service is very simply payment for services rendered. Traditionally, in a fee for service environment, the patient selects his or her physician, the physician provides treatment and recommended follow-up, and bills are sent to the insurance company, who then pays the physician. The patient may be responsible for a deductible charge. Fee for service plans have been typical of private insurance policies that individuals may purchase through a number of insurance providers and are also referred to as private indemnity plans. There are no pre-set limits on benefits, as long as services are "reasonable and necessary" as determined by a physician's order and provided by a qualified provider. In defining reasonable and necessary services, qualified providers, and need for continued treatment, private insurers typically follow Medicare or Medicaid guidelines, which are described later in the chapter.

## Managed Care Organizations

Managed care refers to the management of and controlled access to medical resources in an effort to control costs that escalated secondary to a predominance of fee for service plans, which allowed health care costs to escalate. Managed care is a term that refers to a variety of methods of cost containment. They vary in levels of cost-containment measures initiated through beneficiary rules such as use of a primary care physician, network of physicians, point of service, or limitation of specialty services. All of these plans usually include a primary care physician, who is seen as the "gatekeeper" of all further provision of services. Many plans identify the type of physician included in the plan. Point-of-service plans allow for more flexibility in choice of physician or service providers.

The following are types of managed care:

### HEALTH MAINTENANCE ORGANIZATIONS

The HMO designates a list of physicians who are contracted as primary care physicians (PCP). The PCP is the patient's principal doctor, and any referrals for other health care services must be made through the PCP, unless otherwise stated in the patient's plan. The goal of regulating the use of specialists and other health care professionals is to contain health care costs by limiting utilization of specialists. An occupational therapist or OT facility must be designated by the HMO as a provider of occupational therapy in order to be eligible for reimbursement of services.

Under an HMO, hospitalization or number of therapy visits will be authorized over a given time frame or for a specific number of visits. Frequently, the number of visits authorized initially is few and any additional authorization is required for additional visits. Under these plans, co-payments are required.

### PREFERRED PROVIDER ORGANIZATIONS

This is a reimbursement method in which an insurance company establishes a group of preferred health care providers, including physicians, hospitals, and other professionals. These providers have agreed to pre-determined reimbursement rates or methods. The

Table 5-1

## *Reimbursement Terminology*

| TERM | DEFINITION |
|---|---|
| Co-payment | The amount a patient pays per visit or episode in conjunction with that paid by the insurance provider. |
| Qualified provider | A health care professional who is deemed appropriate to provide treatment for a given condition. "Qualified" is frequently determined by the Medicare guidelines of "skilled" or "non-skilled." |
| Skilled | A health care provider who has met certain educational credentialing requirements and provides intervention at a certain level of complexity. Interventions themselves may be classified as skilled. |
| Non-skilled | A health care provider who does not meet the educational and credentialing requirements of a skilled provider and provides intervention according to guidelines designated by the skilled practitioner. Interventions themselves may be classified as non-skilled. |
| Entitlement program | A program of funding health care that covers certain groups (that are "entitled" to benefits) based on criteria that may include age, type of condition, or services required. |
| Prospective payment system (PPS) | A term referring to a system of payment that pre-determines payment for health care based on a set of pre-determined criteria. DRGs and the RUGS III system (see below) are examples of prospective payment systems. |
| Diagnostic-related groups (DRGs) | A classification of a condition, based on demographic criteria such as diagnosis, age, gender, other existing medical conditions that is used to determine the type, amount, and duration of treatment that will be reimbursed. A patient is categorized based on these demographic factors and reimbursement for services is determined accordingly. |
| Tax equity and financial responsibility rates (TEFRA) | Limited Medicare Part A reimbursement by establishing DRGs. Established guidelines for rehabilitation units and reimbursement in rehabilitation units. |
| Primary care physician (PCP) | A physician designated by a managed care company who serves as the "gatekeeper" of medical services. The use of the PCP contains medical costs by regulating visits to specialists and other health care professionals. Services not referred by the PCP are not eligible for reimbursement. |

continued

*Table 5-1 continued*

### Reimbursement Terminology

| TERM | DEFINITION |
|------|-----------|
| Rehabilitation diagnosis | A diagnostic category that qualifies a patient for re-imbursement for services in a designated rehabilitation unit. |
| Fiscal intermediary | A third-party payer designated to process claims for government programs, such as Medicare. |
| Individual education plan (IEP) | A plan indicating goals, recommended intervention methods, and progress of children and students receiving services under IDEA. It is generally a collaborative effort between parents, teachers, and health care providers. |

Adapted from Pallister, J. (1996) *Dictionary of business*. Oxford: Oxford University.

patient receives the maximum benefit when he or she uses a preferred provider organization (PPO). The PCP is considered the "gatekeeper" of the patient's care. A PCP referral is often required and some plans allow referral for services by a specialty physician. The occupational therapy provider must be a member of the PPO network to maximize coverage and avoid out-of-pocket expenses for the patient. The services of non-PPO providers or out of network providers may be covered at a percentage. Verification with the insurance company or pre-authorization may be required and there is often a limit on number of visits or a cap or the amount of reimbursement.

## Capitation

Capitate plans, or capitation, refers to reimbursement that is determined statistically and that allocates a pre-determined amount of money to the primary caregiver per beneficiary. Anticipated costs are determined by national and regional data. The health care provider receives a pre-determined amount per patient member, per month, whether members do or do not access care. In other words, if a physician sees 100 patients from a managed care organization, the physician will be allotted a set amount of money, per patient, to provide care. The physician receives the payment regardless of patient utilization. The philosophy is that this will be an incentive for the physician to provide only truly necessary care.

# Guidelines for Reimbursement

Guidelines for reimbursement come from varied sources including state and federal guidelines, accreditation agencies such as the Joint Commission on the Accreditation of Hospitals (JCAHO), Commission on Accreditation of Rehabilitation Facilities (CARF), national certification, state licensure requirements of qualified providers, and standards of practice.

## *Prospective Payment Systems*

A prospective payment system (PPS) is one that sets legislated guidelines and limits for payment of services prior to the time service is rendered (prospectively). In prospective payment systems, the health professional knows in advance the amount of funding available based on certain criteria and must tailor intervention to meet these limits in a cost effective and medically sound manner. Diagnostic-related groups (described below) are a form of PPS, as are the resource utilization groups (RUGS) classifications defined by the Balanced Budget Act of 1997.

## *Diagnostic-Related Groups*

A diagnostic-related group (DRG) applies to a patient in an in-patient setting to determine the rate of reimbursement. DRGs emerged in the 1980s as a cost-containment measure as hospitals were mandated by Medicare to assume a prospective payment system in 1984. Factors such as primary and secondary diagnoses and demographic criteria such as age, gender, other existing conditions are used to determine the type, amount, and duration of treatment that will be reimbursed. A patient is categorized based on these demographic factors, and reimbursement for services is determined accordingly. Cases that fall outside of the prescribed guidelines are called outliers and application may be made for extension of reimbursement benefits.

## *Tax Equity and Financial Responsibility Act*

The Tax Equity and Financial Responsibility Act (TEFRA) served to expand limitations on Medicare Part A, which covers inpatient care. As part of this legislation, TEFRA guidelines for rehabilitation units and reimbursement were established.

# Medicare/Medicaid

Medicare is a federally mandated health insurance program formed as a result of Title XVIII of the Social Security Act, expanded by the Johnson Administration in the 1960s. This is an entitlement program for persons 65 years or older, certain people with disabilities, and people with permanent kidney failure who are treated with dialysis (CMS, 2002). The services such as those identified above are considered in the accepted standards of medical practice to be "a specific and effective treatment of the patient's condition" (2002) and are determined by current research in the medical field. In other words, intervention that is supported to be a sound intervention for a particular condition is eligible for reimbursement. Medicare is administered by the Centers for Medicare and Medicaid Services (CMS), formerly the Health Care Finance Administration (HCFA). It is available to those individuals who have contributed to the Social Security System for 36 quarters.

Medicare benefits are classified as Part A and B, with each covering separate benefits. Part A covers inpatient therapy or, as termed by CMS, "hospital insurance." Part B covers outpatient services. These benefits are paid according to the DRGs in acute care hospitals or the present TEFRA rates in inpatient acute rehabilitation. Those rehabilitation units in hospitals that are rated at the TEFRA rate require a certification as a Rehabilitation Unit. Once certified, the Medicare requirements of the unit are:

- Admissions are limited to the 10 primary rehabilitation diagnoses
- 75% of the patients must receive 3 hours of therapy at least 5 days a week
- There is documentation of the patient demonstrating progress toward functional goals

Part B is considered the "medical insurance" of Medicare and covers outpatient and home care. By 1986, occupational therapy was included as a free-standing Medicare Part B benefit. Medicare Part B benefits reimburse outpatient therapy and medical services at 80% of charges. Many seniors carry additional secondary or supplemental policies. The requirements of the secondary policy must be followed to allow for coverage of the remaining 20% or the patient is liable for the remaining 20%. Recently, the federal government has been encouraging HMOs or other managed care insurance organizations to provide the supplemental benefits under Medicare.

*[handwritten margin note: Supplemental insurance pays 90% of remaining 20%]*

As with other rehabilitation benefits, Medicare requires a plan of care certified by a physician in order for services to be covered. Services must be provided while the patient is under the care of the physician, the services need to be "reasonable and necessary" to the treatment of the patient's condition, and there is a positive "expectation of change."

## Documentation and Medicare

Documentation requirements for reimbursement through Medicare must relate to reasonable and necessary intervention, the documented plan of treatment, progress in treatment, and discontinuation of treatment.

Medicare guidelines also define whether a service is of a level of complexity to be provided by a "skilled "or "unskilled" provider. CMS determines if the level of service required for payment is "skilled" if treatment can only be performed by a experinced physician or therapist. Occupational therapy personnel must ensure that the services they provide fall into the "skilled" category as defined by Medicare and are documented according to terminology recommended by Medicare guidelines. "Non-skilled" services must be provided by aides in order to be reimbursed and must also be documented as such, also using appropriate terminology as defined by Medicare guidelines (CMS, 2002).

Medicare guidelines state that for reimbursement, intervention must be provided with an expectation that the condition will improve significantly in a reasonable period of time and that improvement is related to restoration of potential. The amount of frequency and duration of treatment must be reasonable.

The plan of treatment must contain the diagnosis, type, amount, frequency, and duration of services to be performed. The plan of treatment should contain anticipated rehabilitation goals what are objective and measurable, have a timeframe, and relate to function. The rehabilitation plan must document:

- An "at least" clause (states minimal expectations)
- The patient's goals for rehabilitation
- Involvement of family and/or significant others, when appropriate
- Rehabilitation goals related to activities of daily living (ADLs), learning, and working
- Measurable criteria and timeframes for achieving goals
- Factors that may influence goal achievement
- Long-term rehabilitation goals
- Short-term rehabilitation goals

Goals must be written in functional terms and developed collaboratively with the patient and family. The measures of rehabilitation goal attainment, successful role performance, changes in level of functioning, efficiency of support resources, and possible barriers should be documented. The plan should identify criteria for transition to less restrictive environments, need for support in the environment, and interventions to reach reasonable goals. Documentation should also include the patient's treatment choices, response to interventions, progress toward goals, and changes in condition.

Goals should take into consideration the patient's activities in areas of self-care, work, and leisure, as well as their expected environment. The patient should be involved in goal-setting. If the goals are preventative, then they need to relate to the patient's medical condition. The patient must show progress toward these goals and, if not, a revision of the plan of treatment needs to be documented. Medicare has denied payment of therapy services when they have been provided to maintain a state of health (e.g., range of motion or strength).

The discontinuation of services is identified when the patient has achieved functional goals, when there is no longer a reasonable expectation of change, and upon reaching a "maintenance" level of care. Establishment of and training caregivers for a "maintenance" program is a covered service. The discharge summary must include a summary of therapy treatment goals. A summary must include the patient's current functional level, the need for continued therapy services or aftercare, and potential for independence.

The federal government administers the Medicare Program under the General Accounting Office (GAO) and is therefore subject to legislative initiatives. A review of the history of health care management in Chapter 3 illustrates the effects of legislation on Medicare. In recent years, health care reform has been seen as a national issue as part of the former Clinton administration in response to escalation of costs and the widely held public perception of the high cost of health care. In addition, there were widely publicized reports of Medicare fraud. The Health Care Finance Administration, in response, requested that the Justice Department vigorously investigate and prosecute reported cases of fraud. Congress responded by instituting progressive budget cuts. The Balanced Budget Act (BBA) of 1997 was passed to enforce a schedule of Medicare cuts. Several amendments (BBA; Public Law 105-33) have had and continue to have significant influences on the practice of occupational therapy.

Subsequent legislative initiatives, such as the Medicare Improvement and Protection Act of 2000 and the Balance Budget Refinement Act of 1999, continue to affect practice. Under such legislation there was a restoration of funding to hospital, inpatient rehabilitation nursing homes, and other providers. These acts lifted the therapy reimbursement caps per calendar year per beneficiary and delayed implementation of the prospective reimbursement for home health services. The CMS must develop as alternative recommendation for congressional action to replace the cap and still control cost growth while assuring appropriate access to care.

## Medicaid

Medicaid is a federal insurance program administered by each individual state, which is designed to serve eligible low-income persons. Title XIX of the Social Security Act provides medical assistance to individuals and families with low income and limited resources. It is a jointly funded venture between the federal and state governments to assist the states in the provision of medical care to eligible persons. An individual is determined eligible by the state and must follow the state statutes for coverage of services. Many states are in the process of enrolling recipients into managed care plans, approved by the state for Medicaid. The eligibility of services may be limited by factors such as the requirement for U.S. citizenship and to be at or below a specific financial status, which may limit enrollment by the working poor.

Similar to the Medicare program, a physician's referral or prescription is required. Preauthorization may or may not be necessary. Re-enrollment periods may also be required.

# State Regulations

Each individual state has guidelines related to the provision of health care. This takes the form of licensure laws and certification of facilities. To qualify for reimbursement under numerous programs, facilities must meet state requirements. Some state practice acts define the occupational therapist's scope of practice and continuing education requirements, which directly affect reimbursement, as the practitioner must meet the requirements to allow the facility to comply with state regulations.

Supervision practices also relate to reimbursement issues. Supervision of COTAs varies from state to state and is dependent on personnel regulatory requirements. In many cases, there is regulation of the OTR, but none of the certified occupational therapy assistant. While the AOTA Model Practice Act makes recommendations on the supervision of assistants and aides (AOTA, 1999) and this can serve as a model, state practice acts determine supervision requirements (Fowler, 2001). This, of course, changes along with legislative activity, and an individual practitioner needs to be aware of these initiatives.

State regulators are interested in the certification of service providers such as those providing services in skilled nursing facilities and home health agencies. These providers undergo regular review of credentialing of professionals to determine if qualified providers are employed. State surveyors may also specifically review organizations due to reported incidents of abuse or neglect of patients. Reimbursement is directly related to the proper credentialing, supervision of health care providers, and ethical practice.

# Federal Guidelines

There are federal guidelines for numerous services that contribute to the health, safety, and general protection of the public. To get an idea of the myriad of federal guidelines, the reader is encouraged to do an Internet search for "Federal Guidelines." The results are amazing—and interesting! General guidelines relating to qualified provider, physician's order, and a written plan of treatment, as seen in the following examples of federal guidelines, pertain to health care and occupational therapy practice:

- 482.56: The hospital provides rehabilitation, physical therapy, occupational therapy, audiology, or speech pathology services; the services must be organized and staffed to ensure the health and safety of patients.
- 482.56a2: Physical therapy, occupational therapy, speech therapy, or audiology; services, if provided, must be provided by staff who meet the qualifications specified by medical staff, consistent with state law.
- 482.56b: Services must be furnished in accordance with a written plan of treatment. Services must be given in accordance with orders of practitioners who are authorized by the medical staff to order the services, and the orders must be incorporated in the patient's record.

# Workers' Compensation

Workers' compensation is a program that is intended to compensate workers for injuries or illnesses incurred due to job-related conditions. Workers' compensation plans are governed at the state level and reimbursement procedures are determined by the state workers' compensation governing body, usually a state board or commission. Policies, therefore, vary by state. Reimbursement for OT services will vary accordingly and practitioners need to be aware of workers' compensation procedures in their individual state. Workers' compensation plans are funded jointly by employers and the state (Thomas, 1996).

COTAs who are employed in outpatient clinics and primarily treat physical injuries are likely to have workers' compensation cases.

# Accrediting Agencies

As occupational therapy educational programs are accredited by the Accreditation Council for Occupational Therapy Education (ACOTE) (see Chapter 4), organizations providing health care are also accredited. While accreditation is technically a voluntary activity, third-party payers may reimburse only for services that are provided by an accredited facility. Recalling that accreditation is a credential that documents adherence to a set of accepted standards, reimbursing services from an accredited institution supports health care of a high caliber. Two of the major accrediting bodies in health care, the Joint Commission for the Accrediting of Healthcare Organizations (JCAHO) and the Commission for the Accreditation of Rehabilitation Facilities, are described here.

## *The Joint Commission for the Accrediting of Healthcare Organizations*

Many hospitals nationwide have chosen to be surveyed by JCAHO. JCAHO accreditation requirements are related to assessment of patients, care of patients, plan of treatment, rehabilitation plan reassessment, and discontinuation of services.

### JCAHO REQUIREMENTS RELATED TO ASSESSMENT

JCAHO specifies the following requirements in order for a facility to meet accreditation requirements. The facility's protocols for assessment and treatment plan (noted below), and other aspects of care must include these criteria. Note that they are in accordance with federal reimbursement guidelines:

- Functional status is assessed when warranted by the patient's needs or condition
- All patients referred for rehabilitation services receive a functional assessment
- Reassessment occurs at regular intervals in the course of care
- Reassessment determines a patient's response to care
- Significant change in a patient's condition results in reassessment
- Significant change in a patient's diagnosis results in reassessment

The care of patients also relates to reassessment. Reassessment includes the extent to which goals are met, improvements in physical dysfunction, reduction in pain associated with movement, orthotic and prosthetic fit and function, as well as patient satisfaction, adjustments to disability, and goal achievement relative to discharge.

### JCAHO Requirements Related to the Rehabilitation Plan

- A rehabilitation plan, developed by qualified professionals and based on assessment of patient needs, guides provision of rehabilitation services
- Qualified professionals implement the rehabilitation; plan with the patient and his or her family, social network, or support system
- Rehabilitation restores, improves, or maintains the patient's optimal level of functioning, self-care, self-responsibility, independence, and quality of life
- The patient's readiness to end rehabilitation services is determined based on written discharge criteria

# Legislation and Reimbursement

The following is a review of the legislation discussed in Chapter 3 with additional information provided regarding the specific guidelines associated with a particular piece of legislation.

Careful monitoring of current legislative issues and activity is possible through state and national professional organizations. AOTA's legislative monitoring organization is the American Occupational Therapy Political Action Committee (AOTPAC), which offers the latest information regarding political activity.

## Omnibus Budget Reconciliation Act (1980)

Prior to the Omnibus Budget Reconciliation Act (OBRA), the home health care benefit was split between Medicare's Part A and Part B and each plan was subject to different coverage and payment requirements. Both Part A and Part B restricted the number of visits to 100, and required that the patient be hospitalized for at least 3 days before being eligible for benefits. In 1980, OBRA relaxed the home health care benefit. The 3-day prior hospitalization requirement and 100-visit limit were removed and for-profit home health care agencies were allowed to become Medicare certified. As a result of report of misuse, in 1997, HCFA mandated Medicare's fiscal intermediaries (FIs) to control utilization. Home health care could now be provided only on a part-time basis (less than 8 hours a day), intermittently (4 or fewer days a week), and to those person's who are "homebound."

Such changes in reimbursement required practitioners to alter treatment priorities and delivery in order to be eligible for reimbursement.

## Tax Equity and Fiscal Responsibility Act (1982)

The Tax Equity and Fiscal Responsibility Act (TEFRA) established the DRGs and affected reimbursement patterns for practitioners in the inpatient setting. Prior to TEFRA legislation and under fee-for-service practices, OT personnel were able to provide care as prescribed by the physician and be reimbursed. Provision of services generated revenue for facility, as reimbursement was available for services as prescribed.

As the first prospective pay system, DRGs significantly altered the reimbursement picture. In order to be reimbursed, physicians and therapists were now required to provide only the services specified by the parameters of a patient's DRG. As a capitated system, there was a set amount of funds allotted per category. The facility kept any remaining funding as an incentive to keep costs down by staying within category guidelines. For example, a facility is allotted $1,500 for a 50-year-old Patient A with condition X based on criteria set in the diagnostic category for patients of this age and gender with this condition. If Patient A's treatment costs total $1,000, the facility keeps the extra $500. If Patient A's care costs exceed $1,500, the facility absorbs the extra expense.

## Americans With Disabilities Act (1990)

The Americans with Disabilities Act (ADA) was passed by Congress in 1990 for equal protection of individuals with disabilities "by extending to them the same civil rights protection guaranteed under the law to people on the basis of race, creed, gender, national origin, and religion." In five titles of the ADA, employment, state and local government services, public accommodation, telecommunications and public accessibility, and transportation are addressed in terms of their accessibility to people with a disability. The creation of this act has afforded occupational therapists with opportunity to establish services related to advocate for their clients in the areas of employment and accommodation of facilities (Kornblau, 2000). As employers, public facilities, telecommunication, and transportation providers are required to comply with the ADA by funding "reasonable accommodations," and funding is prioritized, providing opportunities for reimbursable services for OT personnel.

## Individuals With Disabilities Education Act (1997)

The Individuals With Disabilities Education Act (IDEA) is a reauthorization and extension of PL. 94-142, passed in 1975, which established that each child is entitled to a free and equal education in the least restrictive environment, and that each child would have an individual education plan (IEP). (USDOE, 2002) IDEA broadened services by:
- Expanding mandated services through 21 years of age, versus 18
- Expanding mandated services from birth through age 3 and implementing the use of the individual family service plan (IFSP)
- Changing the term "handicaps" to "disabilities"

Occupational therapy was retained and strengthened as a related service with the assurances of use of qualified providers in the IDEA in 1997. Funding for reimbursement of services became available not only through the school systems, but through state and federally funded programs geared toward early intervention.

This act defines a child with a disability as one needing special education and evaluated as "having mental retardation, a hearing impairment including deafness, a speech or language impairment, a visual impairment including blindness, serious emotional disturbance (hereafter referred to as emotional disturbance), an orthopedic impairment, autism, traumatic brain injury, an other health impairment, a specific learning disability, deaf-blindness, or a multiple disabilities, and who, by reason thereof, needs special education and related services" (Muhlenhaupt, 2000).

The availability of funding through IDEA demonstrates how legislation can open markets for occupational therapy. Reimbursement trends are part of defining settings where OT personnel may find a niche.

## Balanced Budget Act of 1997

Public policy makers passed the 1997 Balanced Budget Act (BBA), which mandated prospective payment systems for SNFs, home health care, and rehabilitation facilities, and required a legislative proposal on a prospective payment system for long-term hospitals. The change from a retrospective payment system to a prospective payment system for post-acute care represented a major policy reaction to the rise in expenditures.

The BBA mandated establishment of prospective payment (PPS) for SNFs effective July 1998, home-health care effective October 1999, and rehabilitation facilities effective October 2000, although the dates have been subject to revision. It also required a PPS proposal for long-term care hospitals by October 1999. Since that time, there has been a delay in the implementation of some of these PPS systems including rehabilitation facilities. This bill radically changed the delivery of occupational therapy services to these populations by placing a $1,500 cap on occupational or physical therapy, combined with speech therapy per beneficiary, per calendar year under Part B of the bill. Due to concerns raised by health care advocacy regarding accessibility to appropriate care, the Balance Budget Refinement Act of 1999 placed a moratorium on the implementation of the $1,500 cap on outpatient rehabilitation under Medicare until 2002. HCFA was mandated to develop an alternative recommendation for congressional action to replace the cap and still control cost growth while assuring appropriate access.

The PPS system imposed by the BBA classifies the beneficiary of Medicare into a category. The payment rate is determined by the federal government and is dependent on factors including regional data and co-morbidities or complications of hospitalization.

Skilled nursing facilities implement the prospective payment system by using the Resource Utilization Groups III (RUG-III) classification system. Reimbursement for occupational therapy services is determined by the RUG-III classification. Similar to DRGs, the RUG-III system classifies conditions into categories based on level of severity. Each category specifies a predetermined number of therapy minutes to which a patient in that category is entitled. The facility is reimbursed through Medicare for the number of therapy minutes allocated by the RUG-III category.

Evaluation for classification in a RUG-III category is done using the minimum data set (MDS) assessment instrument. The MDS is used with patients in transitional care units (TCUs) or SNFs. The MDS combines medical information and current functional status to determine the level of care needed for a resident in a facility. This, in turn, provides justification for reimbursement. The MDS is considered a preliminary assessment and screening of resident problems, and the addition of resident assistant protocols (RAP) makes up a comprehensive assessment. RAP provides a method of identifying problems, triggers for further evaluation, and guidelines to assist in evaluation of 18 most common problems or conditions occurring in patients or residents. For example, RAP 5 is the ADL/functional rehabilitation potential RAP:

- Identifies a problem, such as the inability to perform ADLs (such as self-care)
- Identifies indication for rehabilitation and the potential to improve
- Provides guidelines upon which clinical judgments are based when determining the cause of dependence, the expected course, and which services are indicated

This limited the reimbursement for treatment provided in SNFs and TCUs, and had a direct impact on the provision of occupational therapy services.

The prospective system for HHAs was introduced in October 2000; reimbursement by Medicare was switched from fee for service to a capitated rate under the PPS.

The Outcome and Assessment Information Set (OASIS) is the standard assessment tool that must be used in the evaluation of home health patients. For recertification of Medicare benefits, the home health patient must be recertified per OASIS data, therefore, data is collected using the OASIS every 60 days if the patient requires additional services.

Acute rehabilitation units are the next settings to fall under a similar prospective payment system. The major elements are a patient assessment instrument, patient classification system, a case-mix formula, and payment rate (Kurlander, 2000).

## Medicare, Medicaid, and State Children's Health Insurance Program Benefits Improvement and Protection Act of 2000

This legislation extends the moratorium of the $1,500 cap on outpatient rehabilitation services for another year if alternative policy is not established. The caps are scheduled to be reinstated at the beginning of 2003 (Metzler, 2001).

### Occupational Safety and Health Administration (1999)

Several federal initiatives such as the Welfare to Work Legislation, the proposed Ergonomic Standards by the Occupational Safety and Health Administration (OSHA), and the Ticket to Work and Work Incentives Improvement Act of 1999 all have provided opportunities to expand occupational therapy services in the work practice areas (Kornblau, 2000).

The OSHA Ergonomics Program Standards were not implemented but were designed to "reduce the number and severity of musculoskeletal disorders (MSDS) caused by exposure to risk factors in the workplace" (OSHA, 1998). These standards would have mandated employers to develop a ergonomics program, to respond to employee MSDS reporting, have access to a health care professional, define work restrictions including time off from work, and to provide evaluation and follow up of the MSDS incident. The ergonomics program would have been required to include an evaluation of the effectiveness of the program. Critics pointed to the high costs of implementation of ergonomic programs and the requirements to comply with the standard. Businesses with more than 10 employees would have been required to comply by the January 2001, and those with fewer than 10 employees by January 2005 (Somers, 2001). These guidelines would have opened significant opportunity to occupational therapy practitioners. Although these particular guidelines were not implemented, they are noteworthy for their ability to illustrate how legislation can serve to support occupational therapy practice and its revenue streams. This circumstance validates the importance of occupational therapy's involvement in the legislative and political systems as related to reimbursement issues.

# Reimbursement and Documentation

The purpose of documentation is primarily related to reimbursement and is also important for regulation, risk, or legal and team communication.

A general rule for successful reimbursement emphasizes thorough documentation of patient progress in terminology that demonstrates progress toward functional goals, regardless of payment source. Documentation in the medical record, as well as on federally mandated forms, needs to be included in the patient's record. Medical necessity was the previous guideline for reimbursement, however federal and state reviewers are now looking for medical and functional progress. Additionally, patient participation in the goals of treatment is highlighted.

Documentation is often used to determine the medical necessity of treatment with the premorbid function compared to current function. Anticipated length of treatment, the potential of the patient to benefit from treatment, the patient's actual benefit and improvement in function, and whether treatment fell within guidelines and standard protocols are also expected to be included in documentation. The previous section regarding the Medicare guidelines serves as the standard for documentation in most service areas and will apply to most third-party payers.

Table 5-2a

## Documentation and Reimbursement

| SETTING | REQUIRED DOCUMENTATION | PURPOSE |
|---|---|---|
| SNFs and TCUs | MDS and RAPs | A standard assessment that rates a resident based on medical history, current statutes, and function. MDS scores on a scale from 0 (independence) to 4 (total dependence). |
| Home health agencies (HHAs) | OASIS | Standard assessment tool required by home health agencies. |

Table 5-2b

## Documentation and Reimbursement Timetable

| SETTING | ITEM | TIMEFRAME |
|---|---|---|
| SNFs and TCUs | 1. Initiation of MDS | 1. Within 24 hours of admission |
| | 2. Treatment plan | 2. Completed within 72 hours |
| | 3. Comprehensive assessment | 3. Completed within 5 days and submitted in 7 days |
| | 4. Assessment data are locked in | 4. Within 14 days |
| | 5. Comprehensive care plan | 5. Completed within 21 days |
| | 6. Periodic assessment | 6. Between day 31 and 60, and day 61 and 90 |
| Home Health Agencies (HHAs) | 1. Initial assessment following referral | 1. Within 48 hours |
| | 2. Completed assessment | 2. Within 5 calendar days |
| | 3. Reassessment | 3. Every 60 days |

Very specific documentation requirements are in place for certain types of service delivery such as SNFs, including transitional care units (TCUs), subacute care units, and HHAs. Tables 5–2a and b summarize required documentation and forms according to service delivery areas.

In addition to documentation of assessments, certain language must be used in order to qualify for reimbursement. Again, terminology will change with the times, and it is necessary that the OT practitioner remain apprised of changes in this area. Table 5–3 lists terminology that is acceptable to be used by OT personnel, according to Medicare guidelines.

Table 5-3

## *Medicare Accepted Terminology*

*THE FOLLOWING LIST OFFERS EXAMPLES OF WORDING THAT WILL SUPPORT REIMBURSEMENT.*
*FAILURE TO USE ACCEPTED TERMINOLOGY MAY RESULT IN DENIAL OF REIMBURSEMENT.*

| | |
|---|---|
| Evaluation | Activity analysis |
| Compensatory technique education for ADLs | Adaptive technique education for ADLs |
| Energy conservation | Arthritic techniques/joint protection |
| Work simplification | Environmental adaptation |
| Independent living skill re-education | Neuromotor re-education for ADLs |
| Postural control re-education for ADLs | Sensory retraining |
| Therapeutic strengthening | Progressive ADL re-education |
| Safety education | Therapeutic stretching activities |
| Activity tolerance for ADLs | Functional mobility training for ADLs |
| Positioning for ADLs | Splint application/assessment/adjustment |
| Adaptive equipment analysis/training | Bed mobility training |
| Home program education | Body mechanics training |

In the event a claim to a third-party payer is denied, a facility will generally re-submit the claim with a justification letter intended to clarify any questions raised by the original claim. This is a lengthy and time-consuming process and delays payment to the facility, thus interrupting a revenue stream. Although the entry-level COTA will probably not be responsible for writing a justification letter, knowledge of appropriate documentation guidelines and terminology will help avoid the need for one, serving both the patient and facility more efficiently.

Documentation in the medical record is critical in the event it was to be used in a court preceding. For risk and legal reasons, if something is not documented in the medical record, then it did not occur. If standard occupational therapy practice is followed and tracked by complete and detailed documentation in the medical record, the chance of legal risk is lowered.

Finally, the importance of the medical record cannot be underestimated as a way of communicating to other providers of care. Team member communication from physician, physical therapy, speech language pathology, recreation therapy, social services, case management, and other professionals is important for team collaboration on goal setting and consensus of opinion for treatment planning. Additionally, discharge planning and deposition can be ascertained from the medical record. The general mechanics, clinical elements, and ethics of effective documentation should be understood by students at this point in their education and have probably been practiced in labs and on Level I Fieldwork. In professional practice, the student/COTA should learn their facility's specific guidelines for documentation as related to reimbursement, as they are likely differ somewhat between settings.

# The Business of Finance

The health care business is different than other types of business practices in that there are factors that affect people's health and well-being influencing the basic operation. The industry is regulated by many organizations, both voluntary and involuntary, and the benevolent aspect of the business will always influence its daily delivery practices. Additionally, the reimbursement system is somewhat artificial. What is billed is not always what is paid for, and different rates for the same services or discounts muddy the waters greatly. Health care finance does however adhere to similar basic guidelines of a comparison of revenue (billed versus collected) and operation expenses to create a budget.

Budget principles and finance can be better understood if you apply them to your own household budget. Everyone does some pre-planning (e.g., your income versus your costs for rent or a car) and investing for the future (e.g., buying your car), while realizing that at some point your outlay will be larger than the balance (e.g., you want to take that Caribbean vacation, but don't have the money). Similarly, when an organization builds a budget, it is based on its previous experience or years past, objectives and financial goals for the future, and restrictions due to costs or other factors.

## Determining Budgets

Budgets determine a road map to plan and coordinate activities, evaluate performance, and authorize actions within a defined scope.

Financial accounting is the process of maintaining information about the financial resources, obligations, and activities of an organization. Accounting practices will vary between facilities, but all procedures and statements must conform to generally accepted accounting principle (GAAP) as defined by the Financial Accounting Standards Board. Financial benchmarks are overall guiding objectives that provide a framework for budget development. Operational targets are made by determining expense and revenue balances throughout the year. The income statement provides a record of revenue and expenses. This affords an opportunity to monitor the budget and change allocation of funds as necessary.

Budget is determined by the sources of income to an OT department and generally includes third-party reimbursement and other sources of funding specific to a particular service delivery setting. Expenses include capital expenditures and operating costs such as salaries, supplies, overhead, and depreciation of equipment. These will vary depending on the practice setting.

Stated simply, budgets are determined by anticipating revenue, usually based on past experience and performance of a department, and assessing revenue against projected costs. Obviously, the department will want to show profit, and the budget (usually expenditures) will be adjusted to anticipate an acceptable profit margin.

Again, each setting will have a slightly different process, as well as different revenue sources and costs. The entry-level COTA will become familiar with those relevant to his or her practice setting.

## Types of Budgets

One aspect of budgeting with which the entry-level COTA may be involved is that of establishing priorities for capital and operational budgets. The two types of budgets are discussed below.

### CAPITAL

A capital budget is the amount of money that an organization or department allocates to large equipment that is intended for use over an extended period of time. A general guideline is items that cost over $300, and lasting longer than a year comprise the capital budget, although the exact numbers may vary between settings. Examples of capital expenditures in an OT clinic might be a stove or refrigerator.

### OPERATIONAL

The basic operational budget consists of revenue and expenses that occur on a daily basis. For example, revenue may include volume projections for activity or patient services. Operational expenses are items that are used in the provision of services. Frequently, these are expendable items and supplies. An example might include evaluation forms, splinting materials, or cooking supplies.

COTAs, who are primarily responsible for delivery of service, are directly involved with supplies, equipment, and other resources used on a daily basis. Therefore, your first involvement with budget as a COTA might be to make suggestions and assist in determining priorities for operational and capital budgets.

## Other Factors Influencing Budget

The need to be profitable in the health care climate of managed care, capitation, and prospective payment systems such as DRGs and RUGs has influenced staffing patterns in OT service delivery settings. Although at entry-level, the COTA is not likely to be involved in determining staffing patterns, an understanding of the process may be helpful.

In a fee-for-service reimbursement system, OT is a service that generates revenue, as third-party payers reimburse for a percentage of services recommended by a physician. Staffing patterns are determined by patient/client need, and OT personnel is staffed to meet the demand. In this system, providing more services is profitable.

Conversely, in a capitated or prospective pay environment, the level of reimbursement is predetermined. The facility receives a set amount of dollars based on criteria discussed earlier in this chapter from which they must show productivity (profitability). In this situation, provision of services represents an expense. Staffing patterns must be maintained at a level that supports productivity, and the demand for personnel may drop.

A staffing plan states both the number of staff and type of staff (COTA, OTR, or aide) needed to provide care. The OT manager will determine a staffing pattern based on client/patient population needs and the types of services to be provided in the setting. The manager must also consider the mission and organizational goals of the facility. Services must be of acceptable quality as well as cost-effective. Managing the staffing component of the budget requires clinical knowledge, a knowledge of funding and reimbursement regulation, and an application of judgment and ethics.

## Common Financial Terminology

An understanding of terminology that is common to accounting procedures is necessary to understand the business aspects of an OT department. Table 5–4 defines common financial/accounting terms.

Table 5-4

## *Common Financial Terminology*

THIS IS COMMON TERMINOLOGY THAT IS ENCOUNTERED IN THE BUSINESS WORLD. THE COTA
MAY ENCOUNTER THESE TERMS IN THE PROCESS OF PARTICIPATING IN BUSINESS OPERATIONS IN
PRACTICE.

| | |
|---|---|
| Operating budget | A forecast of the financial requirements for the future trading of an organization, including its planned sales, production, and cash flow. |
| Capital | The total value of the assets of a person less liabilities. |
| Capital budget | The sums allocated by the organization for future capital expenditures. |
| Profitability | The capacity or potential of a project or an organization to make a profit. |
| Profit | For a single transaction, the excess of the selling price of an article or service being sold over the costs of providing it. |
| Liquidity | The extent to which a company's assets are liquid, enabling it to pay its debts when they fall due and also to move into new investment opportunities. |
| Liquidation | The distribution of a company's assets among its creditors and members prior to its dissolution. |
| Income | Any sum that a person or organization receives either as a reward for effort or as a return on investments. |
| Revenue | Any form of income. |
| Billed revenue | The amount charged for a service, visit, or procedure. |
| Collected revenue | The amount reimbursed or collected from a service, visit, or procedure. |
| Billed unit of service | The amount of time spent on the performance of the service or procedure recorded for productivity reasons. |
| Depreciation | The diminution in value or a capital asset due to wear and tear or obsolescence over an accounting period. |
| Return of investment or return of capital employed (ROCE) | The accounting ratio expressing the profit of an organization for a financial year as a percentage of the capital employed. Profit is usually taken as a profit before interest and tax, while capital employed refers to fixed assets plus circulating capital minus current liabilities. |
| Operating profit or loss (margin) | The profit or loss made by a company as a result of its principal trading activity. This is arrived by deducting its operating expenses from its trading profit or adding its operating expenses to its trading loss; in either case, this is done before taking into account any extraordinary expenses. |

Adapted from Pallister, J. (1996). *Dictionary of business*. Oxford: Oxford University.

# Billing Procedures

In discussing financial considerations, the importance of proper coding according to the patient's diagnosis cannot be underestimated, as third-party payers base their decisions on diagnostic codes when reviewing files. The COTA who is responsible for completing billing paperwork will need to be familiar with current coding practices. Current resources are important to keep track of the latest changes in diagnostic codes, as correct codes may make the difference in whether or not the facility is reimbursed. An updated ICD9-CM codebook is the standard resource for updating to current coding practices (ICD 9 Code). Additionally, keeping updated on changes through the CMS Federal Register and newsletter publications are helpful.

The typical 10 rehabilitation diagnoses mentioned earlier in this chapter and the ones that are used on the inpatient rehabilitation units are considered standard. The more specific the code, the greater the possibility of reimbursement. For example, indicating whether the patient has a dominant or nondominant hemiplegia as a result of a cerebral vascular accident can greatly affect function, and, therefore, will be related to reimbursement.

Specific service codes are used to bill for occupational therapy services under Physician Medicine and Rehabilitation. For Part A Medicare these codes are called HCPCS codes and are generally numbered from 97001 to 97799 (Medicare Part A Newsletter, 1998). Certain codes are viewed by HCFA intermediaries as reimbursable, however this does change yearly and is "clarified" frequently. The occupational therapy provider must be updated through current publications. Most codes are time related in 15-minute increments.

The codes used for workers' compensation do vary according to the state regulations or an individual insurance plan. Many times these payers follow the Medicare guidelines and utilize ICD 9 CM, CPT coding, or HCPCS rules.

# Fiscal Responsibility

Budget principles include profitability (operating margin), liquidity (cash on hand), and capital structure (with devaluation or depreciation costs). The relationship of debt to fund balance or maximum annual debt service coverage may be a target for fiscal accountability. A business may choose three times the coverage as its target.

Productivity standards refer to the amount of time a practitioner is engaged in billable activities, such as patient treatment. Productivity standards for therapists have been used in many practice environments. These guidelines change according to the setting the therapist is practicing in and the financial targets of the organization. Productivity standards of 60% to 75% may be considered to be the average (Kurtz, 1999).

# Managing Limited Resources

At a time when controlling costs is a concern, effective management depends on leadership and supervision skills, financial accountability based on objective measures, and tracking outcomes of care.

Leadership, as discussed in Chapter 1, plays a role in managing limited resources. With the changes in the reimbursement patterns that ultimately affect practice, OT personnel have been and will continue to be called upon to respond positively and creatively to change. The leadership skills that allow us to discover new directions and to grow in fresh professional directions allow us to respond positively to regulatory changes.

In addition to the discussion on leadership that was presented in Chapter 1, there are two additional leadership theories that warrant mention. Transformational leadership theory, discussed by Burns (1978) and later by Bass (1985), may be important to review in the current climate of health care. Transformational leadership traits during a time of transition are considered an effective form of leadership versus the transactional leadership. The transactional leader provides the incentive for workers by exchanging rewards for performance. The performance is rewarded for agreed upon objectives and the manager will not intervene unless the objectives are not being met. A transformational leader is one who motivates followers to work for transcendental goals and for higher level self-actualizing needs instead of working through simple exchange relationships with followers. Self-reinforcement rather than external rewards motivate followers (Reiss, 2000).

Described as a leadership style that includes idealized influence-attributed; idealized influence-behavior; inspirational motivation; intellectual stimulation; and individualized consideration, this style of leadership fits well with occupational therapy leadership needs in the current financial climate of health care.

Financial accountability through an objective system of evaluating fiscal performance is important in a time of change. Based on this record of performance, sound financial decisions can be made. Occupational therapy services are labor intensive and require resources in manpower. This determines the majority of the costs and because of this reason, staffing is critical.

Management can focus on efficient methods of staffing, staff development, and interdisciplinary or transdisciplinary approaches for optimum utilization of resources without compromising quality of care. Regulations and ethical considerations do prevent over utilization of therapy assistants and aides.

Outcome tracking can be utilized for measuring an organization's overall performance or by an individual case-by-case basis. Outcome tracking is simply monitoring performance to ensure effectiveness of services and fiscal accountability. Quality management techniques, discussed in Chapter 8, are a formalized method of outcome tracking. The Functional Independence Measure (FIM) has been used as the standard for evaluating the patient's performance over their time in rehabilitation. Contribution to the national database provided by the Uniform Data System (UDS) also details how your organization performs in relation to other rehabilitation facilities. Development of outcome data can also be done on a case-by-case basis or by evaluating each patient's progress in rehabilitation. Evidence-based practice, which is designed to guide everyday practice by utilizing critical thinking skills when examining a clinical question, can enhance the outcome tracking process. It is a "conscientious, explicit, and judicious use of current best evidence in making decisions about the care of individual patients and should also include a cost considerations. The practice of evidence-based means integrating individual clinical expertise with the best available external clinical evidence from systematic research" (Sackett et al., 1997). Occupational therapists need to become clinician-researchers to evaluate clinical evidence and apply it to their patients, residents or clients. The mechanics of carrying out research are addressed in detail in Chapter 9.

# Summary

The COTA, although mainly concerned with provision of service, is also part of the business operations of their department and facility. To effectively serve in this role, the COTA must have a general understanding of financial considerations.

The challenge for health care providers in the current climate of change and transformation is to determine the standard of care acceptable that coincides with the greatest possible outcomes of care at the lowest cost. In keeping with this challenge, OT personnel must be cognizant of reimbursement processes and the regulations by which they are governed. Federal and state legislation and guidelines, type of payment system, accreditation requirements, effectiveness of documentation, and elements of business all influence whether a facility is reimbursed for the services provided by practitioners. As a COTA, part of the responsibility you assume is to understand and apply these elements to achieve a cost-effective department that also delivers quality care.

Leadership skills will enhance the COTAs ability to effectively adapt to an ever-changing fiscal environment in health care. The reader is referred back to review Chapter 1, with an emphasis on recognizing opportunity in times of change.

Finally, the reader is reminded that nothing in this aspect of health care is static. Regulations change with legislative sessions. Procedures change with health care organization mergers. The examples offered here are just that—examples. Know your facility and its specific requirements and stay current, as regulations and do differ across time and practice settings.

# References

American Occupational Therapy Association. (1999). Guide for supervision of occupational therapy personnel in the delivery of occupational therapy services. *Am J Occup Ther*, 53, 592-597.

Balanced Budget Act. (1997). Pub. L 105-33, 42 C.F.R. $410.59 et seq.

Bass, B. M. (1985). *Leadership and performance beyond expectation.* New York: Acedemic Press.

Burns, J. M. (1978). *Leadership.* New York: Harper and Row.

Centres for Medicare and Medicaid. (2002). *Skilled Nursing Facility Manual.* Retrieved November 20, 2002, from http://cms.hhs.gov/manuals/12_snf/SN00.asp

Fowler, R. J. (2001). Are you following your state's supervision regulations? *OT Practice*, 6(4), 29.

Kornblau, B. L. (2000, December). The future of OT work practice. *Work Programs Special Interest Section Quarterly*, 14, 1-2.

Kurlander, S. (2000) Exposing the fine print: HCFA unveils the per discharge PPS for inpatient rehab hospitals and rehab units. *Rehab Economics*, 8(7), 80-81.

Kurtz, L. A. (1999). Creating realistic productivity standards. *OT Practice*, 4(4), 26-31.

Liu, K., Gage, B., Harvell, J., Stevenson, D., & Brennan, N. (1999). Medicare's post-acute care benefit: Background, trends, and issues to be faced. Retrieved August 28, 2002, from http://aspe.hhs.gov/daltcp/reports/ mpacb.htm

Medicare Part A LMRP Newsletter. (1998, February 17). *Health Care Finance Administration Medicare/Medicaid.*

Metzler, C. A. (2001). Participate and communicate. *OT Practice*, 6(2), 8.

Muhlenhaupt, M. (2000). Occupational therapy services under IDEA 97. *OT Practice*, 5(24), 10-13.

Occupational Safety and Health Administration. (1998). *Prevention of work-related musculoskeletal disorders, Item 1218-AB36-2222, Unified Agenda.* Washington, DC: Author.

Pallister, J. (1996). *Dictionary of business.* Oxford: Oxford University.

Quiroga, V. A. M. (1995). *Occupational therapy: The first 30 years 1900-1930.* Bethesda, MD: AOTA.

Reiss, R. G. (2000, June). Leadership theories and their implications for cccupational therapy practice and education. *OT Practice*, 5(12), CE1-CE8.

Sackett, D. L., Richardson, W. S., Rosenberg. W. M., & Haynes, B. R. (1997). *Evidenced based medicine: How to practice and teach EBM.* New York: Churchill Livingstone.

Somers, A. (2001). The gamble on ergonomics standard. *Advance for Occupational Therapy Practitioners, 17.*

Thomas, V. J. (1996). Evolving health care systems: Payment for occupational therapy services. In AOTA (Ed.), *The occupational therapy manager.* Bethesda, MD: AOTA.

U.S. Department of Education (2002). *IDEA '97 Regulations.* Retrieved November 18, 2002 from, www.ed.gov/offices/OSERS/Policy/IDEA/regs.html

# Bibliography

American Occupational Therapy Association. (1922). Minutes of the fifth annual meeting. *Archives of Occupational Therapy, 1, 232.*

American Occupational Therapy Association. (2000). Occupational therapy and the Americans with disabilities act (ADA). *Am J Occup Ther, 54,* 622-625.

Americans With Disabilities Act. (1990). Pub L. 101-336.42 U.S.C. 12101. Retrieved August 28, 2002, from http://www.usdoj.gov/crt/ada/ pubs/ada.txt

CARF: The Rehabilitation Accreditation Commission. (2002). *Home page.* Retrieved November 4, 2002, from www.carf.org

Centers for Medicare and Medicaid Services. (2002). *Home page.* Retrieved November 4, 2002, from www.cms.hhs.gov

Cusick, A. (2001). The experience of clinician-researchers in occupational therapy. *Am J Occup Ther, 55,* 9-18.

Federal Guidelines For Hospitals. Rev 103. A-103–A-107.

Federal Register. (1999). *Medicare program; Prospective payment system and consolidated billing for skilled nursing facilities-update; Final rule and notice. Schedule for calendar year 2000; proposed rule (HCFA-1913-F).* Retrieved August 28, 2002, from www.access.gpo.gov/su_docs/aces/aces140.html

Federal Register. (2002). *Database for the 1995, 1996, 1997, 1998, 1999, 2000, 2001 and 2002 Federal Register* (Volumes 60, 61, 62, 63, 64, 65, 66 and 67). Retrieved November 4, 2002, from Federal Register Online via GPO Access :www.access.gpo.gov /su_docs/aces/aces140.html

Goode, C. J. (2000). What constitutes the "evidence" in evidence-based practice? *Applied Nursing Research, 13*(4).

Individuals With Disabilities Education Act Amendments. (1997). Public Law 105-17, U.S>C> www..ed.gov/offices/OSERS/IDEA/frnotice.html.

Individuals With Disabilities Education Act Amendments. (1997, March 12) Public Law 105-12, Final Regulations, 34 CFR, parts 300, 303. *Federal Register, 64*(48).

Johnson, K. V. (2000). Home health PPS: The new payment methodology. *OT Practice, 5*(18), CE1-CE8.

Joint Commission on the Accreditation of Health Care Organizations. (2002). *Home page.* Retrieved November 4, 2002, from www.jcaho.org

Kirschner, C. G. (1994) *Physician's current procedural terminology* (4th ed). Chicago: American Medical Association.

Kornblau, B. L. (1999). The ethical and legal implications of the use of aides in occupational therapy practice. *Administration and Management Special Interest Quarterly, 15,* 1-4.

Medicare: The Official U.S. Government Site for People with Medicare. (2002). *Home page.* Retrieved November 4, 2002, from www.medicare.gov

Miller, A. (1998, April 6). Playing by the rules in rehabilitation. *Advance for Health Information Professionals*, 14-17.

New York Public Library. (1998). *New York Public Library Business Desk Reference*. New York: Wiley and Sons.

*Pocket RAP guide for the minimum data set*. (1995). Natick, MA: Eliot Press.

Thomas, J., Lloyd, L., & Hostetler, H. (2001). Capital briefing: New 2001 CPT codes. *OT Practice*, 6(3), 8.

United States Department of Labor: Occupational Safety and Health Administration. (2002). *Home page*. Retrieved November 4, 2002, from www.osha.gov

# 6

# PERSONNEL CONSIDERATIONS AND SUPERVISION

*Sue Berger, MS, OTR*

"I just put on what the lady says. I've been married three times, so I've had lots of supervision."
*Upton Sinclair, 1988*

## Introduction

There is an old joke that goes something like this:
"My boss does bird imitations."
"Oh, he does?"
"Yeah… he watches me like a hawk!"
Although in many situations people have equated supervision with a boss who watches and directs their every move, we will see that in the professional world of occupational therapy (OT), supervision carries a meaning far different from this one. In this chapter, we will examine several descriptions of supervision, as well as the definition put forth by the American Occupational Therapy Association (AOTA). In all instances, we will see that supervision implies a situation of mutual respect, learning, and professional growth.

This chapter will present foundations upon which the new certified occupational therapy assistant (COTA) can establish his or her first supervisory relationship as an occupational therapy practitioner. You will learn the responsibilities of the supervisor and supervisee, factors that guide the frequency and intensity of supervision, and circumstances that contribute to a productive supervisory relationship. In addition, you will be exposed to a variety of methods for advancing your own professional development.

You are encouraged to apply the ideas presented in this chapter in establishing yourself as an OT practitioner. Supervision is a complex and fluid process involving many variables from psychological, communication, leadership, and management theories. If you develop an interest in supervision, leadership, and management, you are encouraged to pursue these areas to enhance your supervision skills and experiences.

# Skills You Will Apply

In learning and developing the skills of supervision, it will be helpful to review and apply skills that have been discussed in previous chapters. Please also refer to Chapter 7 on communication. The current chapter (and others) is intended to present a context into which you can apply communication skill development.

## Leadership and Management

One of the themes that recurs for both supervisors and supervisees is the need to balance the ideals of leadership and the more day-to-day tasks of management. As a supervisor, one must motivate and inspire those they supervise to achieve and maintain passion for what they do. In addition, the supervisor has an obligation to ensure that the responsibilities of the supervisee's position are carried out effectively. Likewise, the supervisee has the responsibility to remain motivated toward growth and professional development and must complete the tasks that allow them to fulfill their commitment to patients/clients and professional colleagues. Understanding the importance of, and the relationship between, leadership and management will assist the practitioner in understanding when each is important in the supervisory relationship.

## Professional Organizations

The AOTA publishes numerous documents on supervision and professional roles and the responsibilities associated with each. In addition, and as we will see in this chapter, state practice acts and other regulatory bodies and guidelines can influence the supervision process. Both supervisors and supervisees are responsible for understanding these guidelines and functioning according to their stipulations. Also, when one has questions about guidelines in supervision, the appropriate professional organization can provide clarification.

## Ethics

As in all professional endeavors, practicing ethically is of paramount importance to the OT practitioner. Supervision is no exception. Concepts of confidentiality, tolerance, veracity, and acting in the best interest of others are all considerations when providing and receiving supervision.

## Communication

Although the chapter on communication follows the chapter on supervision, you are encouraged to think ahead to the communication practices that would enhance the supervision process. Methods of providing feedback, giving constructive criticism, styles of listening, assertiveness and tact, and the way in which we attend to the emotional processes of ourselves and others play a significant role in supervision. The reader is encouraged to view this chapter on supervision as one of the many contexts to which communication strategies can be applied.

Occupational therapy assistants work in a variety of settings with a variety of professionals. Before one can fully understand supervision, one must learn and understand the roles and educational backgrounds of those who supervise occupational therapy assistants (occupational therapists) and those who occupational therapy assistants supervise (other occupational therapy assistants, aides, volunteers, and students). Only then will individuals be able to work together as a team to best benefit the client. Therefore, this chapter will first address educational backgrounds and job responsibilities of occupational therapists, occupational therapy assistants and aides and then explore information about professional growth and development focusing on supervision and mentorship.

# Educational Background of Personnel

Beginning in January 2007, all occupational therapy entry-level programs need to be at the master's degree level of academic preparation. Therefore, all entry-level occupational therapy practitioners will have a minimum of a master's degree. Occupational therapists who graduate with a baccalaureate degree in OT prior to the transition of academic program to master's level will be allowed to continue to practice without being required to pursue a post professional degree, though this may be encouraged by individual places of employment. Therefore, practicing OTs may hold a(n):

- Baccalaureate degree in OT (and have graduated prior to implementation of new guidelines)
- Entry-level master's degree in OT (e.g., a baccalaureate degree in another major and a master's degree in OT)
- Post-professional master's degree in OT (e.g., a baccalaureate degree in OT and a master's in OT)
- Doctorate in OT

Whatever the degree, the registered occupational therapist (OTR) has met certain criteria for them to be able to sit and pass the national registration exam. To sit for the exam, all OTRs must have graduated from an accredited OT program, including going through a minimum of 6 months of Level II Fieldwork. Finally, to practice in most states, OTRs must be licensed within that state and therefore meet specific state criteria (e.g., continuing education requirements—see Chapter 4).

COTAs have graduated from an accredited occupational therapy assistant (OTA) program and have gone through a minimum of 16 weeks of Level II Fieldwork, per the 1998 Standards for an Accredited Occupational Therapy Assistant Education Program (AOTA, 1998). If the COTA graduated under the 1991 Essentials for an Accredited Occupational Therapy Assistant Education Program (AOTA, 1991), he or she will have completed a minimum of 12 weeks of Level II Fieldwork. OTAs graduate with an associate's degree in occupational therapy and are then eligible to sit for the national certification exam. To practice occupational therapy, they must also pass the certification exam and be licensed in the state they practice in, if required.

To work as an occupational therapy aide or rehabilitation aide, no specialized academic degree is required. Most facilities require a high school diploma or equivalent and provide training specific to the job.

As a COTA, working closely with an OTR and/or OT aide can be a wonderful learning opportunity and facilitate dynamic, progressive, and effective OT interventions.

Personality, OT philosophy, environment, and knowledge can all influence whether an OTR/COTA/OT aide team will be effective. Understanding the individuals with whom one works will be one step toward a positive relationship and effective OT intervention. The reader is referred to Chapter 7 (Communication) for strategies relating to building effective professional interpersonal relationships. Goleman's (1998) principles of emotional intelligence and emotional competency are especially relevant in the interpersonal process and can play a large and positive role in the outcome of professional and supervisory relationships. In understanding the individuals, it is important to also understand the job responsibilities of the OT personnel with whom one works and be able to identify areas that overlap and areas that are distinctly separate.

# OT and OTA Roles

The OT practitioner functions in a variety of roles including clinician, consumer educator, fieldwork educator, supervisor, administrator, consultant, fieldwork coordinator, faculty, program director, researcher, scholar, and/or entrepreneur (AOTA, 1993). In any of the above roles, the OT or OTA can be functioning at an entry, intermediate, or advanced level.

Traditionally, occupational therapists and occupational therapy assistants begin practice as entry-level practitioners and then progress to higher levels of practitioner before moving on to other roles. The major role of the OTR practitioner is to "provide quality occupational therapy services, including assessment, intervention, program planning and implementation, discharge planning-related documentation, and communication. Service provision may include direct, monitored, and consultative approaches" (1993, p. 1088). The major function of the COTA practitioner is to "provide quality occupational therapy services to assigned individuals under the supervision of an OTR" (1993, p. 1088). The role delineation documentation from AOTA was developed and written in 1993. The Commission on Practice has begun to review and update these roles to better meet the needs of the profession. The information included here is what is documented by AOTA as of this writing. For a more in-depth representation of this information, the reader is referred to www.aota.org/members/area2/docs/sectionb.pdf.

Although Table 6–1 elaborates on the role differentiation between the entry-level OT and OTA practitioners, in today's changing health care environment and with emerging practice areas, an occupational therapist or occupational therapy assistant's first job may be that of consultant, entrepreneur, or almost any of the roles mentioned earlier. Many OTs and COTAs have developed new positions for themselves because of newly acquired knowledge in program development, marketing skills, and the ability to seek supervision independently. These are just some of the skills needed to find, develop, and choose exciting job positions.

In some of these new roles, the guidelines for supervision a COTA may be less clear, and questions may arise. For example, in a setting where a COTA is not acting "officially" as a COTA, but is using OT skills and expertise, what are the guidelines for supervision?

There are also situations where a COTA who has been practicing for an extended period of time is faced with being supervised by a newly graduated OTR or an OTR who is new to a particular setting. In these situations, the COTA, by virtue of experience, may be better versed in that particular setting than the OTR. Yet, the guidelines state (and remain true) that the OTR is ultimately responsible. These cases require good communication, active problem-solving, and creative approaches. Supervision in exceptional situations sometimes requires "out of the box" approaches that are thoughtful and ethical as well.

No matter what role you choose, and in situations as those exemplified in the preceding paragraph, it is important that you function within the AOTA guidelines that pertain to educational background, years of experience, and skill level. At times, a unique approach may be required that utilizes the expertise that is available, yet is within the guidelines and

Table 6-1

## *Comparison of the Roles of the Entry-Level OTR and COTA Practitioner*

| *OTR* | *COTA* |
|---|---|
| Responds to requests for service | Responds to requests for service, initiates referral as needed |
| Screens individuals | |
| Evaluates individuals | Assists with data collection |
| Interprets evaluation | |
| Develops and coordinates intervention plan, including treatment goals | Develops treatment goals under supervision of OTR |
| Implements treatment | Implements intervention plan under supervision of OTR |
| Adapts environment, tools, materials, and activities | Adapts environment, tools, materials, and activities under supervision of OTR |
| Monitors response to intervention and modifies as needed | Provides direct service following a documented routine under supervision of the OTR |
| Communicates and collaborates with other team members | Communicates with other team members in collaboration with OTR |
| Follows policies and procedures required in the setting | Follows policies and procedures required in the setting |
| Develops home and community programs | |
| Terminates services | |
| Monitors own performance; identifies supervisory needs | Monitors own performance; identifies supervisory needs |
| Documents services and maintains records | Maintains records and documentation under supervision of OTR |
| Maintains treatment area, equipment, and supplies | Maintains treatment area, equipment, and supplies |
| Quality assurance activities | Quality assurance activities in collaboration with OTR |
| Provides in-service education | |
| Professional development | Professional development |
| Schedules and prioritizes workload | |
| Participates in professional and community activities | Participates in professional and community activities |
| Functions according to AOTA Code of Ethics and Standards of Practice | Functions according to AOTA Code of Ethics and Standards of Practice |

Adapted from American Occupational Therapy Association. (1993). Occupational therapy roles. *Am J Occup Ther, 47*(12), 1087-1099.

may involve activities such as additional training or use of a consultant. When in doubt about guidelines, a review of the appropriate AOTA documents can clarify questions that the practitioner may have. In addition, the AOTA Practice Department can further assist in explaining and interpreting guidelines and in exploring problem-solving approaches as necessary.

# Professional Growth and Development

The OT Code of Ethics states "OT personnel shall take responsibility for maintaining competence by participating in professional development and educational activities" (AOTA, 2000). There are many ways to achieve this. Seeking different positions, both laterally and hierarchically, challenges one to learn new and different information. Using supervision and seeking mentorship, attending conferences, continuing education workshops, and taking additional coursework are all appropriate ways to advance professionally. Taking on the role of supervisor and/or fieldwork educator are other ways to stay current professionally. The next section of this chapter will briefly discuss ways of participating in professional development.

# Making the Most of Supervision as a Professional Development Tool

AOTA (1999a, p. 592) defines supervision as "a process in which two or more people participate in a joint effort to promote, establish, maintain, and/or elevate a level of performance and service. Supervision is a mutual undertaking between the supervisor and the supervisee that fosters growth and development; assures appropriate utilization of training and potential; encourages creativity and innovation; and provides guidance, education, support, encouragement, and respect while working toward a goal."

There are a number of ways to structure supervision to gain as much as possible from the experience. MacRae (1998, p. 68) suggests that "face-to-face supervision that is structured, regular, consistent, and process-oriented helps to establish a solid basis for the exchange of information and timely problem-solving." Ryan (1998) suggests the use of performance criteria, reciprocation of ideas and problem-solving, periodic assessment of professional competency and growth, and regular meetings in which these elements can be addressed. General supervision practices that can provide a strong foundation for these activities to occur include:

- *Setting a designated and prioritized time for a supervision meeting.* While this may seem difficult in the hectic health care settings of today, the benefits of establishing consistent communication can actually save time in the longer term. A well-prepared supervision session, achieved by applying the steps that follow, can be conducted in 30 minutes per week, with informal communications occurring in the interim.
- *Having a written agenda.* Time allotted for supervision can be more effectively used when both supervisor and supervisee come to the session knowing their issues of priority. This can be accomplished by keeping a running list of supervision topics as they occur during the week. Jotting these down on a pad of paper is an efficient way to do this. Items can be prioritized so that the most pressing issues are sure to be addressed.

- *Actively participating in the supervision process on both the supervisor's and supervisee's parts.* Specific methods for implementing communication processes that contribute to successfully addressing the following supervision topics will be addressed in Chapter 7. General communication topics that are considered critical to benefiting from supervision include actively evaluating and discussing levels of competency and exploring methods for professional development and growth, setting performance-related competencies and methods of achievement, as well as seeking and providing feedback regarding performance and the professional development process.

- *Maintaining records of professional development.* By keeping records of goals, areas for development, and professional achievement, both supervisor and supervisee are able to observe progress and make adjustments to job expectations as needed. In addition, continuous records facilitate the performance review, which generally occurs on an annual basis and sometimes more frequently for new staff. This also enables the performance review to be a summary of overall performance, with no unexpected feedback present in the formal evaluation. MacRae (1998) emphasizes that "surprises" detract from the evaluation and that they should not occur. In other words, the formal performance evaluation should include only issues that have been addressed in regular, ongoing supervision.

In the subsequent sections, specific responsibilities of the supervisor and supervisee in achieving successful supervision will be addressed.

# Providing Supervision—The Role of the Supervisor

The number of hours and amount of on-site supervision are not the only factors that determine effective supervision. Quality is as important as quantity; and to provide and receive quality supervision, one needs to be dependable, attentive, respectful, collaborative and reflective (Hanft & Banks, 1999). Open communication is required to be able to implement these traits. To begin any supervisory relationship, one must acknowledge each other's expectations of the supervisory process. MacRae (1998) suggests that desirable supervisor traits that contribute to open communication include enjoying working with people, possessing strong interpersonal capabilities, having a genuine concern for those with whom they work, setting clear expectations, and serving as a role model. MacRae also emphasizes that the supervisor should have a clear understanding of his or her supervisory style. Supervisory styles are discussed later.

An effective supervisor needs to have a sound knowledge base (and more importantly, know how to access information as needed); be able to provide constructive criticism, encouragement, and positive feedback appropriately; and be optimistic and open toward a supervisory relationship. These are addressed in Chapter 7.

Clearly, a supervisor must possess a strong knowledge of the technical skills needed in a specific area of practice in order to facilitate the skills of those they supervise and to ensure quality of care to the patients or clients they serve.

Ryan (1998) also emphasizes the need for the supervisor to conduct supervision with a strong understanding of the requirements set forth by state practice, AOTA guidelines, and other regulatory standards. (It is also the responsibility of the supervisee to maintain a current knowledge in these areas.) In addition, the supervisor must achieve a balance between the managerial and operational concerns with the more inspirational focus of providing leadership. MacRae (1998, p. 65) refers to this balance as "the ability to enable, educate, and administer."

# Receiving Supervision—The Role of the Supervisee

Though OTRs sometimes work without supervision, a COTA, as required by AOTA, must be employed under the supervision of an OTR. Being the recipient of supervision is not a passive job. To be able to benefit from quality supervision, one must possess many of the same skills needed to provide quality supervision. Being able to be sensitive, dependable, attentive, respectful, collaborative, and reflective are all requirements of both an effective supervisor and supervisee. In addition, as a supervisee, one needs to be able to apply and integrate knowledge and information, accept feedback (both positive and negative), and be open to new ideas and change. Open communication is key to enabling any supervisor/supervisee relationship to work.

As a supervisee, one needs to clearly state one's needs and wants. Paramount to achieving this is the ability to engage in self-reflection and understand one's own learning style, strengths and weaknesses, goals, motivators, and the type of support and direction one needs in various situations. It is the supervisee's responsibility to communicate these elements to the supervisor. One must come to supervision open to gaining new insight, ideas and strategies to be an effective practitioner. In addition, it is up to the supervisee to let the supervisor know, in an assertive and tactful manner, if supervision needs to be provided in a different style. In other words, if supervision needs to be offered more regularly, if feedback needs to be done in a different manner, or if there is some other element that requires modification, the supervisee must communicate his or her needs.

As stated previously, it is also the supervisee's responsibility to understand the requirements of their state practice act, AOTA guidelines, and other regulatory standards such as those set forth by Medicare and other agencies. The supervisee must bring any perceived discrepancy in any of these areas to the supervisor's attention and be prepared to address any concerns from both ethical and legal perspectives.

It is also to the supervisee's advantage to maintain a record of supervision sessions, topics discussed, and goals set and met, as well as copies of performance reviews. Documentation of continuing education activities can be a strong asset in the professional development process. Particularly in the case of the COTA working toward accomplishing service competency, records of achievement can be a valuable tool. Maintaining your own file of pertinent records may serve you well by providing a readily available record of your qualifications in the event of a new job, change of supervisor, or other professional transition.

The best supervisory relationships occur when both parties come into the relationship hoping to grow professionally and personally from the experience, aware that there is always more to learn, and that a supervisory relationship is not a one way relationship. Communication goes in both directions as does the learning and benefits of being a supervisor and supervisee. No one is too old or too experienced to benefit from supervision, and no one is too young or too "green" to have nothing to offer a supervisory relationship.

# Standards and Styles of Supervision

Quality supervision is key to both professional growth and providing best practice occupational therapy. Quality includes the manner in which supervision is provided, the sensitivity displayed toward individual needs and differences, and awareness of the general environment.

Table 6-2

## AOTA Levels of Practice

| LEVEL OF PRACTICE | NUMBER OF YEARS OF PRACTICE |
|---|---|
| Entry | Less than 1 year |
| Intermediate | 1 to 3 years |
| Advanced | 3 or more years |

Adapted from American Occupational Therapy Association. (1999a). Guide for supervision of occupational therapy personnel in the delivery of occupational therapy services. *Am J Occup Ther, 53*(6), 592-594.

Table 6-3

## AOTA Supervision Guidelines

| LEVEL OF SUPERVISION | AMOUNT OF SUPERVISION |
|---|---|
| Close supervision | Daily, direct contact |
| Routine supervision | Direct contact at least every 2 weeks with interim supervision as needed |
| General supervision | Direct contact at least every month with interim supervision as needed |
| Minimal supervision | On an as-needed basis |
| Continuous supervision | Direct, on-site supervision at all times |

Adapted from American Occupational Therapy Association. (1999a). Guide for supervision of occupational therapy personnel in the delivery of occupational therapy services. *Am J Occup Ther, 53*(6), 592-594.

As mentioned, there are regulatory guidelines that influence the supervisory process. AOTA provides guidelines for supervision of the OTR, COTA, and OT aide, but it is important to be sure to meet state licensure laws and reimbursement criteria as well, when considering supervision. For example, the Centers for Medicare and Medicaid (CMS) specifies certain supervision requirements regarding provision of service and documentation by students. In order to be reimbursed by Medicare for services, a facility must abide by the CMS guidelines. In this case, supervision protocols are determined by criteria outside of AOTA requirements. In cases of discrepancy between guidelines, the legal requirements (usually the most stringent) must take priority.

Table 6–2 explains the AOTA definitions of levels of practice, which separate OT practitioners into entry level, intermediate, and advanced, depending on the number of years of practice. Each level has a recommended frequency and intensity of supervision.

The guidelines differentiate levels of supervision as close, routine, general, minimal, and continuous, determined by the frequency of contact, as shown in Table 6–3.

Table 6–4 clearly delineates AOTA guidelines for the amount of supervision required, and whom the OTR and COTA can supervise. Again, state, federal, and third-party reimbursers often dictate more stringent or different requirements. One must follow the strictest

Table 6-4

## Guide for Supervision of Occupational Therapy Personnel

**Type of Supervision For:**

| | OTR | COTA | AIDE |
|---|---|---|---|
| Entry-level therapist | Recommended: Close supervision | Required: Close supervision | For client-related tasks: Continuous supervision; other tasks as determined by supervisor |
| Intermediate-level therapist | Recommended: Routine or general supervision | Required: General supervision | For client-related tasks: Continuous supervision; other tasks as determined by supervisor |
| Advanced-level therapist | Recommended: Minimal supervision | Required: General supervision | For client-related tasks: Continuous supervision; other tasks as determined by supervisor |

**Supervisory Activities For:**

| | OTR | COTA | AIDE |
|---|---|---|---|
| Entry-level therapist | Supervises: OTAs, aides, Level I students, volunteers | Supervises: Aides and volunteers | No supervisory responsibility |
| Intermediate-level therapist | Supervises: All of the above, Level II students and entry-level OTRs | Supervises: All of the above, Level I OT and OTA students, Level II OTA students, and entry-level OTAs | No supervisory responsibility |
| Advanced-level therapist | Supervises: All of the above and all-level OTRs | Supervises: All of the above and all-level OTAs | No supervisory responsibility |

Adapted from American Occupational Therapy Association. (1999a). Guide for supervision of occupational therapy personnel in the delivery of occupational therapy services. Am J Occup Ther, 53(6), 592-594.

requirements mandated to assure compliance with governing bodies. Keep in mind that supervision is determined not only by the number of years of employment as an OT practitioner, but as importantly, the amount of supervision depends on clinical experience, level of expertise, and roles and responsibilities of the specific job. For example, an OTR who has 15 years' experience working in mental health is not qualified to supervise the clinical activities of neonatal intensive care (NICU) OT staff.

The number of hours and the amount of on-site supervision are not the only factors that determine effective supervision, the style of supervision is also very important. There are several different styles of supervision, yet one individual rarely supervises with one style and rarely does any one individual always benefit most from one style. The skill of knowing what style fits both the situation and the individual being supervised is a skill necessary to be an effective supervisor.

A combination of varying amounts of directive and supportive behavior determines the type and style of supervision. Directive behavior is when a supervisor tells the supervisee what to do, where to do it, when to do it, and how to do it, and then closely monitors the actual performance. Supportive behavior is the process of listening, encouraging, and facilitating the supervisee in decision-making and performance. Though many styles of supervision have been identified, most fall into one of the categories of supervision from the Situational Leadership Model (Wilkinson & Wagner, 1993), which include:

- Directing—high direction, low support
- Coaching—high direction, high support
- Supporting—low direction, high support
- Delegating—low direction, low support

No one style is correct or best. Effective supervision occurs when the supervision style matches the need of the individual being supervised. This is dependent on the individual's knowledge base, motivation level, and learning style along with the specific task, environment, and timeline. Therefore, the same individual might benefit from direct supervision for certain tasks and supportive supervision for other situations. Though it is obvious that the task, timeline, and even environment will change, it is just as common that for a specific task the individual's knowledge base, motivation level, and even learning style might be different. In general, high direction and high support (coaching style) are most appropriate for new graduates, new staff, and those who are changing areas of practice. In other words, when knowledge and experience are limited, this style of supervision is effective. With more experience, less direction and support are needed, and a delegating approach becomes more suitable. Again, this is a very general guideline, and each situation must be evaluated individually, taking numerous factors into account. For example, in the event of an emergency situation, the supervisor might take control and provide high direction to the staff, regardless of experience levels, in the interest of resolving the emergent conditions.

It is helpful to consider the following elements when determining the style one might assume as a supervisor, or request as a supervisee.

## Knowledge Base

Keep in mind whether the individual being supervised is an entry-level, intermediate, or advanced practitioner in the area being supervised (i.e., clinician, faculty member), and whether the academic degree is OTA or OT, along with prior experience and knowledge for the specific task being addressed.

## Motivation Level

Seek out information about what motivates this individual to succeed. For some individuals, increased knowledge and professional growth are the motivating factors. For others, benefits and money are key. For others, a pat on the back or compliment will reinforce positive behavior.

## Learning Style

The adult learner comes with a wealth of knowledge from life experience to build upon. It is important to keep in mind that an adult learner is often motivated to learn because of a desire to grow, thereby having very strong internal motivation (Knowles, 1973). If tasks are assigned that will promote individual growth and increased knowledge and builds upon life experience, then often the adult learner will be inherently motivated to succeed. Years of experience can also influence the content and style of supervision.

## Experience

A new graduate COTA might be looking for supervision in the area of clinical skills, documentation, and guidance with administrative issues such as scheduling and transporting clients to therapy. A COTA with 4 years experience might be looking for guidance with specific treatment strategies along with ideas to facilitate professional growth. On the other hand, a Level I OT student might be hoping to learn the role of the OT in a specific setting along with advantages and disadvantages of working in this environment. Knowing the expectations of the individual being supervised in advance will enable one to make effective use of supervision time, along with learning about his or her knowledge base, learning style, and factors that are motivating to him or her.

# Fieldwork Responsibilities

As an OTA with quality fieldwork experiences, it becomes your professional responsibility to provide quality fieldwork education for others who graduate after you. Once you have been working as a COTA for one year, you are qualified to be a supervisor for OT and OTA students on Level I Fieldwork and OTA students on Level II Fieldwork. It becomes your job to teach others about OT practice. To be an effective fieldwork supervisor, it is important that you:

- Assure open communication and supervision for the student
- Assure that the student receives an orientation to the facility and the policies and procedures of the placement
- Assure that the student receives written fieldwork performance objectives, expectations, and timelines through the fieldwork experience for his or her achievement
- Provide the student with experience with individuals of varying ages, deficits, and delivery models
- Assess skill and knowledge level of the student
- Be familiar with the school's and facility's respective responsibilities, as outlined in a written fieldwork agreement (required by AOTA)
- Maintain communication with the school within the parameters of confidentiality and other ethical and legal parameters

- Provide the student with ongoing feedback along with formal evaluation (AOTA, 1998; AOTA, 1991)

The premises and criteria of successful supervision apply to fieldwork students as well as to certified OT personnel.

All of the guidelines for an occupational therapy fieldwork experience (Level II) and more specific directions for the fieldwork educator can be found at: http://www.aota.org/nomembers/area13/links/LINK06.asp or in *The Guide to Fieldwork Education* (AOTA, 1991). Becoming a fieldwork supervisor is a large responsibility and requires a great deal of effort, but the effort and responsibility lead to much learning and growth by both the supervisor and student. Being a fieldwork supervisor is not only a way to give back to your profession, but also a great opportunity for professional growth.

# Mentoring

A mentor is a combination of a wise advisor, a teacher, and a coach. One way to define mentoring is an "intensive, one-to-one form of teaching in which the wise and experienced mentor inducts the aspiring protégé into a particular, usually professional, way of life" (Parkay, 1988, p. 196). A mentoring relationship goes beyond teaching. First, it develops over time, sometimes years; the relationship is usually deeper and more holistic than a teacher-student relationship; finally, the mentee learns much more than professional knowledge from the mentor (1988). A mentor is one who guides, has gone before, and helps another accomplish his or her goals. A mentee is one who is guided and receives understanding, support, encouragement, acceptance, and concrete help on the way to accomplishing goals.

A mentor:

- Creates an environment of trust, which allows mentees to honestly share their experiences and thoughts
- Provides specific knowledge and/or resources to encourage professional and personal growth
- Encourages a mentee to consider alternate views and opinions
- Acts as a role model and motivates the mentee to take risks, make decisions without certainty of results, and continue to overcome obstacles to reach their goals
- Stimulates critical thinking in regard to professional and personal development (Cohen, 1995)
- Everyone can benefit from a mentor throughout all levels of their professional development

# Seeking Support and Mentorship

A mentor can play an invaluable role in one's professional career and personal life. A mentor does not need to be employed at the same place as the mentee. Sometimes a mentor/mentee relationship is arranged in a formal manner, but more often, a relationship develops before one realizes or even calls the individual a mentor. A teacher, supervisor, colleague, or relative might play the role of mentor. An individual may have many mentors in a lifetime just as one person may mentor several individuals.

Finding a mentor is not an easy task. Personalities must mesh and the mentor must be willing to take the time and energy required to provide support, guidance, and knowledge. When this relationship works, it can be a very positive and satisfying one for both individuals involved.

# Continued Competency

Seeking supervision and mentorship; attending continuing education conferences; and taking additional coursework, providing supervision, developing programs, publishing, presenting, and researching are all ways to advance professionally. In 1997, AOTA approved a formal way to acknowledge COTAs who participate in many of these activities and therefore "achieve advanced levels of practice" (AOTA, 1999b). This acknowledgment is called the OTA advanced practitioner (AP). To become an advanced practitioner, and be entitled to add the initials "AP" after one's name, one needs to meet extensive criteria as listed below:

- Initial national certification as an OTA and state licensure, where applicable
- Minimum of 5 years experience as an OTA
- Minimum of 4 years experience in a specified area of practice within the last 5 years
- Letter of reference from a recent OT supervisor
- Continuing education in a specified area of practice in the last 5 years
- Completion of professional activities that:
  1. Are in the specified area of practice
  2. Have occurred within the past 5 years
  3. Equal a minimum of 50 points, per the AP point criteria (AOTA, 1999b)
  4. Include at least six of the nine categories of professional activities as specified in the AP criteria (AOTA, 1999b)

The requirements to meet the final criterion consist of a large variety of options, including, but not limited to, publishing, presenting, supervising, developing programs, research, and committee participation at state and national levels. The AP credential can be awarded in any practice area in which a COTA has achieved these criteria. Largely, the AP credential can be highly individualized.

Becoming an advanced practitioner is voluntary. Passing the certification exam signifies that one has met the minimum requirements to work as a COTA. Becoming an advanced practitioner indicates that one is truly an expert and leader in a specific area of practice. It is an effective statement that verifies your skills both to yourself and the public.

# Overview of Communication Skills

Though the next chapter discusses communication skills in detail, it is worth addressing them now briefly to emphasize the importance of good communication during supervision. Communication is a skill that can be learned and improved upon. It is a necessary skill for being an effective supervisor and also for being able to benefit from supervision. Communication occurs verbally and nonverbally, both being very important to the message being conveyed.

Giving and receiving feedback is an inherent part of the supervisory process. One needs to be able to give both positive and constructive feedback so that it will be heard and received. Conflict resolution is critical when addressing needs and issues as they arise, as conflict is an inevitable part of any relationship at one time or another.

The next chapter will address these issues and more. Remember, they are key to being not only an effective supervisor, but also to being an effective occupational therapy assistant.

# Summary

Quality supervision is critical toward both a positive client outcome and a meaningful and successful career. To be an effective supervisor, it is important to know the educational background, roles, and responsibilities of the individual(s) you are supervising. Only then can you guide the individual in the best direction possible. As a COTA, you may have the opportunity and privilege to supervise all levels of COTAs along with OTA and OT students at different points during their education. Supporting them and guiding them to becoming skilled practitioners is an extremely rewarding responsibility. It also provides a wonderful opportunity for your own professional growth.

Supervisory responsibilities are only one of the many ways to pursue professional development. Taking courses, reading professional journals, participating in research and other scholarly activities, presenting at conferences, and participating on state and national committees are some other strategies to stay current in an ever changing field. By seeking supervision as needed, along with participating in some of the above activities, you will be able to enjoy a challenging yet rewarding profession while providing high-quality therapy to your clients.

## CASE STUDY

Carol graduated 2 years ago from an OTA program and since then has been working as a COTA at a rehabilitation hospital. She decided she wanted to expand her experience so she took a new job in a school system. She was told she would be working between four elementary schools within the district and that there was one OTR who performs the evaluations for all the children in the district, which includes four elementary schools, two middle schools, and a high school. The district employs four COTAs, one OTR, one registered physical therapist, and five speech and language pathologists. The school is also very committed to educating future rehabilitation practitioners and has an active student affiliation program in all disciplines.

Carol is excited about her new position and is looking forward to learning many clinical skills used in the school setting. Though she feels she has excellent professional and people skills and she did well in her pediatrics course in school, she worries that the one weekly supervisory session will not be enough.

1. How else can Carol get the guidance and learn the skills she needs to succeed at her new job, besides her weekly supervisory meetings?

2. What are some strategies Carol can use to benefit the most from the limited supervision time?

3. What strategies should the supervisor use to meet Carol's needs and assure quality services for the student?

# References

American Occupational Therapy Association. (1991). *Guide to fieldwork education*. Rockville, MD: Author.

American Occupational Therapy Association. (1993). Occupational therapy roles. *Am J Occup Ther, 47*(12), 1087-1099.

American Occupational Therapy Association. (1994). Occupational therapy code of ethics. *Am J Occup Ther, 48*(11), 1037-1038.

American Occupational Therapy Association. (1998). *Guidelines for an occupational therapy fieldwork experience—Level II*. Retrieved August 28, 2002, from www.aota.org/nonmembers/area13/links/LINK06.asp.

American Occupational Therapy Association. (1999a). Guide for supervision of occupational therapy personnel in the delivery of occupational therapy services. *Am J Occup Ther, 53*(6). 592-594.

American Occupational Therapy Association. (1999b). OTA *advanced practice program fact sheet*. Retrieved August 29, 2002, from http://www.aota.org/members/area9

American Occupational Therapy Association. (2000). *Occupational therapy code of ethics*. Retrieved June 8, 2002, from http://www.aota.org/general/coe.asp.

Cohen, N. H. (1995). *Mentoring adult learners: A guide for educators and trainers*. Melbourne, FL: Krieger.

Goleman, D. (1998). *Working with emotional intelligence*. New York: Bantam Press.

Hanft, B., & Banks, B. (1999). Competent supervision: A collaborative process. *OT Practice, 4*(5), 31-34.

Knowles, M. (1973). *The adult learner: A neglected species* (2nd ed.). Houston, TX: Gulf.

MacRae, N. (1998). Supervision. In K. Jacobs & M. Logigian, *Functions of a Manager in Occupational Therapy* (pp. 63-79). Thorofare, NJ: SLACK Incorporated.

Parkay, F. W. (1988). Reflections of a protégé. *Theory Into Practice, 27*(3), 195-200.

Ryan, S. E. (1998). COTA supervision. In S. E. Ryan (Ed.), *The comined volume: COTA (2nd ed.) and Practice issues in occupational therapy*. Thorofare, NJ: SLACK Incorporated.

Wilkinson, A. D., & Wagner, R. M. (1993). Supervisory leadership styles and state vocational rehabilitation counselor jobs satisfaction and productivity. *Rehabilitation Counseling Bulletin, 37*(1), 15-23.

# Suggested Readings

American Occupational Therapy Association. (1999). Guidelines for use of aides in occupational therapy practice. *Am J Occup Ther, 3*(6), 595-597.

Bird, C. A. (1997). A survival guide to supervising a student. *OT Practice, 2*(3), 26-29.

Collier, G. F., & O'Connor, L. (1998). Collaborative supervision, real-life skills. *OT Practice, 3*(4), 46-48.

Dimeo, S. B., Bruns, C., & Malta, S. (1997). A supervision workshop. *OT Practice, 2*(8), 47-48.

Gaffney, D. (2000). How does supervision change as students progress? *OT Practice, 5*(2), 7-8.

Glantz, C. H., & Richman, N. (1997). OTR-COTA collaboration in home health: roles and supervisory issues. *Am J Occup Ther, 51*(6), 446-452.

Youngstrom, M. J. (1998). Evolving competence in the practitioner role. *Am J Occup Ther, 52*(9), 716-720.

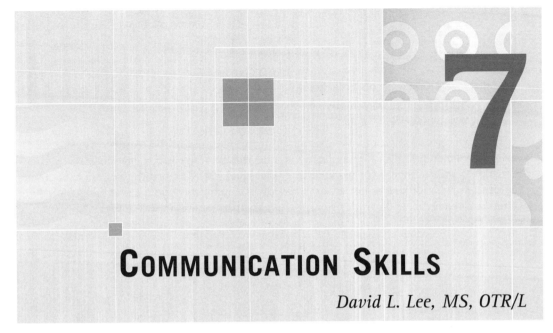

# COMMUNICATION SKILLS

*David L. Lee, MS, OTR/L*

*"To effectively communicate, we must realize that we are all different
in the way we perceive the world and use this understanding
as a guide to our communication with others."*
— Anthony Robbins

## Verbal Communication Strategies for Teamwork and Supervision

As we continue into the 21st century, occupational therapy (OT) practitioners and students are increasingly encountering new issues and situations where they require the skills to understand and effectively deal with differences among people in the workplace. In the most basic sense, verbal communication is an intricate means of dealing with differences among people through the exchange of verbal information. When encountered with a controversial issue, should the practitioner deal with the issue assertively and express their true feelings without violating other people's rights for the sake of the department? Or should the practitioner try to resolve the conflict through a process of negotiation? Through what means or which strategy should he or she resolve the conflict? These issues are pertinent to the occupational therapy practitioner in the context of the modern health care system. Practitioners who move further into leadership positions are required to use their verbal communication skills to execute obligatory management responsibilities in the workplace.

Communication, considered to be the most important managerial skill (Umiker, 1998), is the vital cornerstone to improving teamwork, quality, employee productivity, supervision, and ultimately, health care services. Arguably, good communicators are not born with the skills to negotiate or effectively assert their opinions in order to resolve conflict; communication skills are learned skills.

This chapter describes effective strategies to enhance necessary verbal communication and interpersonal skills for effective supervision and enhanced teamwork, all of which are vital components to the success of the OT practitioner. The verbal communication strategies and approaches include:

- Principles of emotional intelligence
- Principles of effective communication
- Assertiveness skills
- Negotiation and collaboration skills
- Skills for giving constructive feedback
- Conflict resolution skills

This chapter will also examine appropriate technology use in the context of communication, documentation and it implications, and the common issues encountered by the modern OT practitioner in the workplace. This chapter was written with the intent that the OT practitioner will further his or her necessary communication skills for enhanced supervision and teamwork skills in the workplace, with the progression into a supervisory position in the context of the modern health care industry.

# Skills You Will Apply

## *Leadership*

Effective communication is vital to carrying out the role of a leader. In implementing effectual communication practices, the leader consciously practices the communication habits described in this chapter and exercises concepts of emotional competence to select appropriate strategies. The student is encouraged to apply communication processes to developing leadership skills.

## *Management*

In the event that the certified occupational therapy assistant (COTA) assumes a management role, it is likely that supervision of other staff, per American Occupational Therapy Association (AOTA) guidelines and/or state practice act guidelines, will be part of the management responsibilities. Communication with other staff will be of primary importance in informing them about policies, regulatory requirements, standards for documentation and reimbursement, and other clinical task concerns. Applying communication strategies facilitates the supervisory process.

## *Development of Health care Management and Political Concerns*

The COTA or other OT practitioner who becomes involved with political activities or advocacy for the profession will find it necessary to communicate with policy makers at many different levels. By applying concepts of emotional competence and effective communication strategies, the OT practitioner increases their sensitivity to and understanding of policy makers' concerns and their personal ability to advocate for occupational therapy.

# Principles of Effective Communication

A consistency in the modern health care industry is the fact that it is constantly changing (AOTA, 1996; Metzger, 1982; Umiker, 1998). Verbal communication is essential among practitioners and management for continued and enhanced employee productivity and satisfaction, cost-effectiveness, quality, and health care services. The following are underlying principles of effective communication between employees and supervisors that the OT practitioner may consider:

- Effective communication must include a message being sent by the sender and received with "reasonable fidelity" and determination by the receiver
- Communication should be "directional" (e.g., upward, downward, or horizontal) from the sender to the receiver
- Two-way communication may be more effective in that the communication should allow for feedback, such that the sender may:
  1. Know that the receiver has received and understood the message
  2. Learn how to gauge and improve communication with the receiver in the future
- Communication includes a variety of verbal and nonverbal components. Nonverbal communication includes facial expressions, body posture and movements, tone of voice, hand gestures, dress, and actions
- People generally hear, read, and choose to understand only the messages that relate to their own values, interests, needs, and desires
- Communication should not be regarded as a tool or "helping" aspect of the organization; rather, it should be an essence of organized activity and the basic process from which all other functions derive
- Ineffective communication may lead to conflict and wasted time and resources, which leads to decreased productivity and increased costs (Lombardi, 1993; McConnell, 1993; Metzger, 1982; Umiker, 1998)

# The Concept of Emotional Intelligence

The concept of emotional intelligence and emotional competence is based on the work of Dr. Daniel Goleman, CEO of Emotional Intelligence Services in Sudbury, MA. Emotional intelligence is the perception of and sensitivity to both one's own and others' feelings and emotional state; emotional competence is the ability to use a variety of responses and interpersonal skills to respond in a manner that facilitates communication, relationships, and team function (Goleman, 1998). Having gained considerable attention over the last several years, the application of these concepts are credited with ensuring one's success more than technical skills (Cherniss, 2000).

Using Goleman's concepts of emotional intelligence and competence, this section of the chapter will address the importance of applying these themes in the professional occupational therapy setting. They are intended as a framework for applying the skills discussed in the remainder of the chapter.

Using the concepts of emotional intelligence and competency, this chapter will examine communication that the COTA is likely to engage in while in the professional occupational therapy setting. Goleman's (1998) Emotional Competence Framework (applied to OT practice in Table 7–1) provides the foundation for using these concepts, summarizing personal competence as the abilities that determine how we manage ourselves and performance and social competence as the manner in which we handle our relationships.

Table 7-1

## Summary of Emotional Competence Concepts

| EMOTIONAL COMPETENCE SKILL AND DEFINITION | APPLICATION TO THE OT PRACTICE SETTING |
|---|---|
| *Self awareness*: Includes recognizing one's emotions and how they affect others, recognizing one's level of competence, and appreciating one's worthiness and abilities. | The OT practitioner:<br>• Understands one's responses to both team members and clients or patients.<br>• Recognizes and acts in accordance with one's professional boundaries and skill level in practice.<br>• Recognizes one's role as a contributing team member in relation to others. |
| *Self-regulation*: Includes monitoring one's responses and exercising self-control over those that are impulsive or inappropriate, being honest and dependable, being responsible for what one does (or doesn't do), and being flexible and accepting change. | The OT practitioner:<br>• Responds assertively and professionally in the practice setting.<br>• Follows through on practice responsibilities in a manner that speaks to one's accountability.<br>• Responds constructively to the ever-changing practice environment. |
| *Motivation*: Includes working to improve one's skills and to meet high standards, contributing to one's organization or team goals, taking appropriate initiative, and dealing constructively with situations that may appear to hinder one's progress. | The OT practitioner:<br>• Participates in continuing education and meets continuing competency requirements.<br>• Supports the mission and goals of the practice setting.<br>• Takes responsibility for self, behavior, and learning by seeking out and pursuing appropriate activities.<br>• Seeks to find solutions to difficult situations that arise in practice. |
| *Empathy*: Includes recognizing and respecting others' emotional states and viewpoints, seeking to understand and facilitate competent behavior in others based on their level of ability, being sensitive to others' needs, honoring diversity, and understanding and respecting the political structures, emotions, and relationships in a group. | The OT practitioner:<br>• Works in a manner that honors and incorporates team members' feelings and ideas.<br>• Applies OT principles of purposeful activity to supporting the highest level of function in patients or clients and team members.<br>• Applies the OT ethical principle of beneficence in dealing with clients or patients and team members of diverse backgrounds.<br>• Responds constructively to organizational and team group issues. |

continued

Table 7-1 continued

## Summary of Emotional Competence Concepts

| EMOTIONAL COMPETENCE SKILL AND DEFINITION | APPLICATION TO THE OT PRACTICE SETTING |
|---|---|
| *Social skills:* Includes using effective means to persuade others, using effective listening techniques and written or spoken communications skills, resolving conflict through negotiation and other appropriate means, applying leadership principles in the development of others, working well with change, building favorable relationships, working cooperatively, and facilitating group goal achievement by supporting collaboration and cooperation. | *The OT practitioner:*<br>• Is an advocate for the profession, patients or clients, the team, and self by assertively espousing ethical and sound practice. Applies principles of best practice and evidence-based research in practice.<br>• Actively strives to select appropriate conflict resolution methods to most effectively solve problems.<br>• Considers how to best facilitate team members' roles to achieve goals and actively strives to apply leadership skills in practice.<br>• Works collaboratively with team members to achieve the best possible outcomes, honors others' ideas, and shares own ideas in the interest of goal achievement. |

Adapted from Goleman, D. (1998). *Working with emotional intelligence.* New York: Bantam.

# Communication and Emotional Competence

In every interaction, an individual has the opportunity and responsibility to select the communication strategy that is most likely to facilitate good communication. Effective communication involves making this decision based on the people involved, the situation, and the goals you wish to achieve.

Your ability to effectively communicate regarding a topic relevant to your practice setting or to the profession can enhance or conversely, negate your ability to promote your program, resolve a conflict, or provide leadership. Although we all have a preferred style of communication, we can hone skills in all areas to increase communication effectiveness. By increasing our repertoire of communication behaviors, we expand the choices we have to meet a variety of situations. By thoughtfully applying the concepts of emotional intelligence, the communication skills addressed in this chapter can be selected and learned to enhance communication in management and leadership situations.

# Applying Concepts of Emotional Intelligence

With the awareness of the emotional context of a communication, one can select communication strategies appropriate to the situation. By considering the emotional climate and the goals that one wishes to accomplish with the communication, the concepts of emotional intelligence are applied. Following are several strategies that one might use in executing thoughtful communication.

## *Assertiveness*

Assertiveness skills are a necessity for health care practitioners as they develop their effective communication style within the workplace environment from the first day on the job. Without violating the rights of others, assertiveness is the standing up for one's personal rights and expressing those feelings and beliefs in an honest and direct manner (Umiker, 1998).

From a workplace leadership perspective, supervisors are essentially required to run the department and manage their employees, which, for example, includes the responsibilities of delegating tasks to employees, initiating action plans, or resolving possible conflicts both within and outside the department. In the context of the workplace, a lack of assertiveness on the part of the supervisor becomes readily apparent to the employees as being unreliable in the execution of managerial decisions, ranging from simple decisions to complex issues. The supervisor may also be negatively viewed as being easily influenced by others in the manner of being taken advantage by an employee or another manager.

At the practitioner level, having assertiveness skills is essential for the employee to effectively communicate with supervisors and other team members. When encountering a difficult issue at the workplace, the practitioner may choose one of two actions:

1. Let it go and accept the situation
2. Be assertive and do something about the issue through a process of assertion, negotiation, or even conflict resolution (discussed later in the chapter)

On a personal level, difficulty expressing one's true opinion and feelings to other team members reduces one's self-image and self-respect (Umiker, 1998). In order to effectively develop assertiveness skills, the health care practitioner needs to gauge and identify his or her level of assertiveness by asking the following questions:

- Do you often avoid confrontation with others?
- Do you find it difficult to bring up issues during meetings or conferences and hope someone else will raise the same issue?
- Do you often find yourself doing the work of others?
- Do you often feel that others take advantage of you in any way?
- Do you often say "yes" more often than saying "no"?
- Do you say "yes" when you should say "no"?
- To resolve a conflict, do you usually find yourself giving in all the time?
- In the middle of a making a point, do you often allow people to interrupt you?
- Do you tend to start your sentences with negative self-statements (e.g., "Maybe I'm just slow, but...," "I'm sorry, but...," or "This may sound foolish, but...")? (Umiker, 1998)

Finding yourself answering "yes" to the list of previous questions may be an indication for a need to enhance your assertiveness skills. You can increase your level of assertiveness as a health care practitioner with the suggestions in Table 7–2.

The level of assertiveness may be viewed in the context of being both situational and issue-dependent. People often times view "naturally" assertive people as being extroverted, however, even those considered to be introverted may be assertive on issues in which they have a strong opinion, interest, or a conflicting view. Being assertive and taking the initiative does not mean being aggressive or pushy, it means being able to recognize your responsibility to make things happen. Further, it is important to realize that although individual

Table 7-2

### Assertiveness Exercises

| STRATEGY | DESCRIPTION |
|---|---|
| Learn to say "no" | Set your boundaries and limits, however, effective practitioners use their rights wisely and keep an open mind. From the first day on the job, appropriately emphasize that you are a team player and you are making every effort to learn the department, staff, and its policies. As a team player, let team members know your relationship with the team and where you stand in the department in terms of your responsibilities, level of expertise, and your expectations. |
| Role-play | Identify the common issues with which you have difficulty expressing yourself, and practice engaging in various role-playing scenarios with a close friend or confidant such that you are able feel comfortable expressing yourself with specific or recurring issues. |
| Remember that you are a team player | Remember to appreciate the fact that as a team member you have rights and the skills to be in the role of an occupational therapy practitioner. Often, employees want to be liked by everyone in the department, from the managers to volunteers. However, it is important to realize that pleasing everyone is not feasible in every situation and depending on your job description and level of expertise, every practitioner has his or her own set of responsibilities and roles. |
| Attend an assertiveness seminar or workshop | Many businesses and private corporations, not necessarily in the health industry, offer numerous workshops with specific goals in describing the various effective strategies in improving assertiveness skills in the workplace. |
| Read literature or a book on improving assertiveness skills | Many books and periodicals offer effective strategies and role-playing scenarios to improve confidence and enhance assertiveness skills. |

Adapted from Umiker, W. (1998). *Management skills for the new health care supervisor* (3rd Ed.). Gaithersburg, MD: Aspen.

assertiveness may be improved on a personal level, the assertiveness of individual occupational therapy practitioners together may ultimately affect the department as a whole in a positive and meaningful manner.

## Negotiation

Negotiating, often termed as bargaining or collaborating, is an aspect of the workplace that all practitioners will encounter in the rapidly changing health care industry. Common negotiating issues encountered by the OT practitioner include negotiating employee salaries (e.g., a raise) and vacation schedules, cost issues with product vendors, and performance reviews during departmental meetings.

An important characteristic of being an effective practitioner is the ability to negotiate. More and more people want to participate in decisions that affect them, however, fewer and fewer people will accept decisions dictated by someone else (Fisher, Ury, & Patton, 1991). As part of a team whose members are collaborating on common goals and objectives, the OT practitioner needs to develop effective negotiation skills to make sure their opinions and views are considered, suggest fair and rational solutions, and make sound decisions regarding possibly controversial issues in the workplace. Individuals must feel comfortable working together as a team and striving toward a mutually beneficial end (Lombardi, 1993).

To effectively negotiate, it is important to examine the common types of negotiation strategies and describe the advantages and disadvantages of each. Umiker (1998) identified four types of negotiations encountered in the workplace. The first form of negotiation, the "power play," is an approach based simply upon gaining enough power (through connections, money, powerful friends, credentials, etc.) to overwhelm their opponents. Often this authoritarian strategy of dominance is ineffective, as it leads to counter-dominance. Effectively coping with this approach is accomplished by being more assertive and not aggressive, learning not to take negative words personally, and learning to respond to threats and not be intimidated. In any negotiation, there exists the possibility that the opponent will not back down. Negotiation power is often misperceived as being the number of connections one has or how wealthy one is, rather, it is the attractive power of the two parties of not agreeing on terms (Fisher et al., 1991).

A second form of negotiating involves the parties adopting fixed positions on an issue with which both are unwilling to compromise. It becomes a contest of wills rather than a means for problem solving (Umiker, 1998). This ineffective negotiation process forces both sides to focus on a "take it-or-leave it" solution, which leads to both sides being reluctant to back down in order to save their face and self-respect in defending their position on the issue.

Haggling, the third form of negotiating identified by Umiker (1998), involves employees offering options that are only favorable to them. This one-sided strategy often leads to asking for more than they expect to receive and may also lead to promising more than they know they will deliver. This may be an ineffective strategy in that hagglers may give the other party a small offering to create an effect of obligation or make them feel guilty.

The fourth approach, collaboration and value adding, may be the most beneficial and efficient method of negotiation. Essentially, the employee is achieving his or her goals and needs, while also helping the other party achieve theirs. In this win-win approach, rather than seeking concessions from each other, both negotiators add value to the package; the more creative the options are, the more likely a favorable outcome will result (Umiker, 1998). It is recommended that practitioners emphasize this collaborative strategy in any negotiation process.

In preparation for a negotiation, the OT practitioner may consider the suggestions detailed in Table 7–3 for enhancing the negotiation process.

When people find themselves in a dilemma, there are two common strategies that most people tend use: soft negotiation and hard negotiation (Fisher et al., 1991). Wanting a peaceful resolution and focusing on building a relationship with the other party, the soft negotiator wants to avoid personal conflict and is thus willing to compromise readily in order to reach an agreement. However, the soft negotiator may end up feeling negative about himself or herself, and feel that he or she had been taken advantage by the other side.

Table 7-3

## *Suggestions to Enhance the Negotiation Process*

| STRATEGY | DESCRIPTION |
|---|---|
| Prepare your options and list of wishes in writing | Because everyone has different values and interests, make sure you know what you want, what you are willing to concede, and have a fall-back option or alternative goal. |
| Collect all relevant data | Consider the other party's needs and reply to your proposal by collecting data in a concise and understandable manner. Such data may include departmental policies, protocols, and guidelines. |
| Consider various media | In your proposal, you may want to consider using visuals and other media, such as handouts, graphs and charts, or even a computer slide presentation. |
| Take appropriate actions | Write out your action plan. Prepare opening remarks and possible argument topics in order to influence and emphasize the positive aspects of your proposal. Role-play the negotiation process with a close friend or confidant in terms of what you plan to say. |
| Choose an appropriate meeting place and time | Choose an appropriate time and place for the negotiation process. If a department is going through a difficult process (e.g., financial crisis) or undergoing large changes, it may not be appropriate to bring up the issue of raising salaries or vacation scheduling. |

Adapted from Umiker, W. (1998). *Management skills for the new health care supervisor* (3rd Ed.). Gaithersburg, MD: Aspen.

On the other hand, the hard negotiator is determined to win the negotiation and takes the more extreme positions with the intention that holding out longer will fare better. Ultimately, it becomes a contest of wills. However, this may be an ineffective strategy because the relationship between the hard negotiator and the other side may be adversely affected from the long and arduous process. Other typical negotiating strategies fall somewhere in between soft and hard negotiating. The two issues of negotiation are getting what you want from people and getting along with people.

Fisher, Ury, and Patton (1991) identified the method of principled negotiation as an effective strategy for negotiation. Used internationally and in all areas of the workplace, principled negotiation can be applied to the scope of occupational therapy. Being neither soft nor hard negotiation, it is rather a process of combining aspects of the two. Principled negotiation is based on looking for mutual gains whenever possible, and where there is a conflict of interest, the result of the negotiations are based on fair standards. The methods in Table 7–4 follows four basic principles (Fisher et al., 1991).

To summarize the negotiation process, Table 7–5 provides the major steps, with a description, in a negotiation.

Table 7-4

### *The Method of Principled Negotiation*

| PRINCIPLES | DESCRIPTION |
|---|---|
| Separate the *people* from the problem | The "other party" that you are dealing with is a human being also. He or she are just as unpredictable as you are, and has feelings, emotions, and his or her own personal values (e.g., cultural, social, political). Be sensitive to the human emotions that are involved, especially anger, depression, or jealousy. Build toward a working relationship such that it is important to face the problem and not the people. |
| Focus on the *interests, not positions* | Interests are elements such as desires or concerns that motivate people to do what they do and are the bases for their decisions. According to Fisher, Ury, and Patton (1981), the most powerful interests are basic human needs, such as security, economic interests, and well-being. Any breach of these basic human needs may result in a strong opposition or unconscious resistance, dependent on the issue of the negotiation. |
| Invent *options* for mutual gain | Before deciding on what actions to take or what to do, produce a list of possibilities as options. There are always multiple options in any issue, although not all of them will be favorable to both sides. Further, an awareness that extensive time and effort was put into generating possibilities may increase the likelihood that both sides will agree on certain terms or conditions brought out by the list of options. |
| Insist on using objective *criteria* | The result of the negotiation should be based on an objective standard that is clear and concise. Avoid subjective criteria. |

Adapted from Fisher, R., Ury, W., & Patton, B. (1991). *Getting to yes: Negotiating agreement without giving in* (2nd ed.). Boston: Houghton Mifflin.

Anytime in the negotiation process, either party may encounter a negative situation or issue that may affect their decisions in the end of the negotiation. Table 7–6 lists various barriers and negative aspects to a successful negotiation process.

A common negotiation process encountered by the OT practitioner is the issue of vacation scheduling. A practitioner seeks permission to have a week off next month for a vacation with his or her family. However, the supervisor turns down the permission due to tight employee scheduling next month. Following the collaborative approach to negotiating, the practitioner proposes to make up the time by accepting more weekend hours for next month until the vacation time. The supervisor agrees with the proposal. Both of them win.

In comparison to building assertiveness skills, it is not as feasible to practice negotiation skills due to the possible unpredictability of the other party. One needs to have legitimate issues to effectively negotiate. It is important to realize that every negotiation is different in

Table 7-5

## *The Major Steps in a Negotiation*

| MAJOR STEPS | DESCRIPTION |
|---|---|
| Clarify your interests | Speak for yourself, not the other party. Before stating your interests, ask the other party what points of interest are important to them. |
| Focus on agreement | It is important to first focus on agreement, then identify the problem areas. |
| Formulate possible options | It is better to create more options. Don't hesitate to invent creative options. Consider the other party's point of view. |
| Modify options to the point of agreement | Continue the negotiation process even if efforts on your part are unsuccessful initially. Do not be afraid to ask for a break if the negotiation continues for a long time without achieving a result. It may be that the longer the process, the more apparent it becomes to the other party that you are serious on the issue. Sometimes, the longer the negotiation process, the greater the chance that the other party may give in. On the other hand, the other party may become frustrated, and therefore, it is important for the practitioner to use his or her best judgment as to the length of the process and discussion, dependent on the importance and seriousness of the issue. If unable to agree on certain terms, be willing to compromise with a focus on a win-win outcome. |
| Follow-up on positive terms | Compliment each party for their attention and determination to produce a positive outcome after a long and arduous process, or even a short and simple collaboration. |

Adapted from Fisher, R., Ury, W., & Patton, B. (1991). *Getting to yes: Negotiating agreement without giving in* (2nd ed.). Boston: Houghton Mifflin; and Umiker, W. (1998). *Management skills for the new health care supervisor* (3rd Ed.). Gaithersburg, MD: Aspen.

terms of the various issues, size of the parties, and the particular intent. However, the basic premise and elements do not change in a negotiation. Also, it is important to develop an ongoing relationship with your employees, rather than a particular instance of winning a negotiation on a single issue. On a departmental and project level, negotiating is an important and useful strategy in building teamwork, trust, and rapport among your employees. On a personal level, it may enhance your own sense of confidence and self-esteem as a health care supervisor.

Table 7-6

## Barriers Affecting Successful Negotiation

| Barrier | Description |
|---|---|
| The prospect of deteriorating a personal or professional relationship | This is a reasonable and realistic fear in the workplace that may decrease job satisfaction and increase stress in the department. Disagreement in the workplace is real and common. In taking account of the characteristics of people, some may be extremely inflexible and unforgiving, while others have a fear that other people will take advantage of them further. |
| Use of emotion to influence a negotiation | Emotions such as anger, guilt, or crying may be ineffectual and unprofessional in certain negotiations. There also exists the prospect that a negotiator may not be moved by such an emotional approach, and, in turn, may be unwilling to negotiate in the future. |
| Reliance on a team effort to influence the negotiation | Having a group of supporters may negatively portray the practitioner in lacking the skills and ability to handle a negotiation by him- or herself, which may potentially decrease the unity and teamwork in a department. |
| Delaying the negotiation | Usually in a negotiation, it is better to not delay a much-needed action. A delay in the process is unethical, and may increase employee frustration and workplace stress among the employees, and eventually decrease job satisfaction and productivity. |
| Use of secrecy and deceit | Either party may use these tactics. Withholding information or providing false information, respectively, decreases the chance of a favorable outcome in any negotiation. |
| Use of an ultimatum | Unless absolutely necessary, avoid making a threat or deadline unless you are willing to go through with the process (e.g., threaten to walk out of a negotiation, or, for example, saying "This task better be done, or else..."). |

Adapted from Umiker, W. (1998). *Management skills for the new health care supervisor* (3rd Ed.). Gaithersburg, MD: Aspen.

## Giving Feedback

Providing verbal feedback to practitioners is now more important than ever, due to the emphasis on cost control, quality management, customer satisfaction, and team building in the rapidly changing healthcare system (Umiker, 1998). It is a critical element in the two-way communication of supervision. Essentially, it is difficult to really know what you have communicated until you have received feedback. Feedback is a way of giving help; it is essential information provided by others to help the practitioner discover his or her effec-

Table 7-7

## *Feedback Suggestions*

| STRATEGY | DESCRIPTION |
|---|---|
| Provide constructive, honest, and clear feedback | People may take feedback seriously and, thus, it is important to focus on aspects that will improve future performance. It is important that, as practitioners, we are always learning and can always improve. |
| Provide timely and reliable feedback | It is best to provide feedback soon after the performance or behavior, such that the receivers can evaluate themselves while it is still in memory, although the practitioner is free to use or not use the feedback provided. |
| Avoid personal evaluation | Feedback should be focused on the specific task or behavior and not the quality of the individual. This may reduce the chance of a defensive counter-statement on the part of the receiver. |
| Verify perceptions | Each person's perception of other people is different from another's. It is important to always check and verify feedback from a variety of sources to gain a further perspective on an issue. |
| Gauge the amount of feedback | Providing a little feedback is better than not providing any feedback. Generally, more feedback is better, however, it is more important to provide constructive feedback than irrelevant feedback. It is important to provide feedback in amounts that the receiver is able to process. |
| Watch your body language | People are perceptive to nonverbal feedback, such as body language, facial expression, gestures, and eye contact when providing feedback. For example, the inability of keeping eye contact when providing feedback may be perceived by the receiver that the feedback is not completely honest and reliable. |

tiveness as a communicator (Metzger, 1982). Because feedback provides information to the receiver on how his or her verbal communication and behavior appears and affects other people, practitioners need both corrective and confirming feedback. This provides the opportunity for practitioners to gauge their own effectiveness as communicators and the opportunity to improve trust and performance as a team player in the workplace. Table 7–7 has suggestions for practitioners in providing feedback.

## Conflict Resolution

Conflicts in the workplace are derived from the trends of the modern health care industry, including tighter deadlines, increased workloads, increased demand for higher productivity, and fear of layoffs (Umiker, 1998). Conflict in the workplace is inevitable, whether it is antagonism between employees or simply an interpersonal disagreement on an issue (McConnell, 1993). In relation to communication, conflict resolution ability is an important skill for the occupational therapy practitioner to have in order to effectively build teamwork and develop rapport among colleagues, as well as to resolve conflicts in the modern workplace. The inability to resolve conflicts may result in chronic complaining, decline in attendance, morale, and productivity, stress increase, and possibly violence or sabotage (Umiker, 1998) in the workplace.

To effectively deal with conflicts, it is important to identify the causative factors. Conflicts are often multi-layered, in that there may be underlying reasons, which may not always be apparent (Umiker, 1998). Table 7–8 lists major causes of conflict in the workplace.

There are numerous indicators that signal a conflict within a department, and as a practitioner, it is important to identify these symptoms early through observation and instinct, as it can escalate quickly and lead to negative consequences. Table 7–9 offers potential symptoms, causes, and effects on a department due to interdepartmental conflicts (Lombardi, 1993).

Table 7–10 lists strategies for approaching, avoiding, or coping with conflict-producing situations that fall into five general categories (McConnell, 1993; Umiker, 1998) in the workplace.

Generally, collaborative confrontation is the best conflict resolution strategy in depending on the nature and issue of the situation. In preparing for confrontation, it is important to analyze the situation by asking the following questions:

- What is it that I am trying to accomplish?
- What do I think the other person wants? What are his or her goals? What are his or her misperceptions?
- What am I willing to give up?
- What are my weak points or "hot buttons" and what do I do if they are pushed?
- Which strategy should I use? (Umiker, 1998)

Table 7–11 has strategies and techniques in preparing for a confrontation.

To enhance the conflict resolution process, the following are important tips for a collaborative confrontation:

- Avoid sitting directly across from a person, as it invites opposition. Sit next to each other or walk side-by-side.
- Choose an appropriate time and place. Do not attempt to resolve a conflict when either of you are having a bad day or have low self-esteem.
- Open a discussion with a positive and collaborative manner, "Let's resolve this issue so that we are both satisfied."
- Listen attentively.
- Respect and be responsive to the other person's feelings and emotions, yet respond forcibly when necessary. Validate the other person's feelings to clarify the problem and showing care for the other person's feelings and thoughts. Ask validating questions, such as, "You are angry with me because of this, am I right?"
- Focus on points of agreement and work from there. Seek a win-win solution. Avoid ultimatums.
- Stay calm. Avoid raising your voice and using threatening gestures. Do not touch the other person when he or she is angry. When you feel your emotions are escalating, such as anger or anxiety, tell the person and take a break.

Table 7-8

## *Causes of Conflict in the Workplace*

| CAUSE | DESCRIPTION |
|---|---|
| Unclear expectations or guidelines | When practitioners are unsure of what tasks to undertake, how to undertake them, or what outcomes are expected of them, then conflict arises. Also, policies and guidelines within a department or a whole organization may be ambiguous (e.g., sick day policy, salary increases, sexual harassment policy). Clear expectations in supervision can help avoid this type of conflict at the departmental level. |
| Poor communication among employees | Poor communication, attributed to poor listening skills, poor note-taking and memos, or even unclear e-mail messages, results in misunderstandings. On a personal level, distortions and faulty perceptions through miscommunication (e.g., rumors) can deteriorate friendships and rapport among employees. Keep documentation of meetings, messages, and important conversations. |
| Unclear jurisdiction in the workplace | Disputes arise when the level of authority is not clearly understood or implemented. Conflicts often arise over office space, equipment usage, and monetary reasons, such as funding for projects. Written organizational charts and clear written job descriptions document and clarify information in this type of conflict. |
| Individual and professional differences | Everyone has different fundamental beliefs, values, and ideas. When practitioners feel these are compromised, then conflicts arise. In the context of the health care system, disputes also arise between professions, in terms of conflict of interest and disagreements on division of labor (e.g., occupational therapy, physical therapy, speech pathology, nursing, and physicians). Clear but cooperative roles within a setting and a strong professional identity can help in this situation. |
| Changes in the organizational system | Any change in the system, such as staffing or operational changes, may be susceptible to conflict and disagreement. |

Adapted from Umiker, W. (1998). *Management skills for the new health care supervisor* (3rd Ed.). Gaithersburg, MD: Aspen.

Table 7-9

## *Symptoms and Effects of Interdepartmental Conflict*

| SYMPTOMS | DESCRIPTION |
| --- | --- |
| Anger | Loss of temper, lack of patience, or confrontational behavior may be demonstrated in various ways during a conflict. Anger may also manifest itself as apathy. |
| Avoidance/apathy | This symptom, less subtle than anger, may negatively affect teamwork in that an employee avoids contact and declines to work with a specific colleague. This results in unfinished tasks and decreased communication among employees. Over time, this may have negative implications as it leads to the exclusion of other team members in the organization during group processes (e.g., team projects) due to personality conflicts. |
| Blame | Mistakes or poor performance may lead to blaming among employees. This leads to hostility and questionable trust among team members. |
| Excuse making | An employee will use another's behavior as an excuse for not performing their task. A statement used by employees to emphasize negative traits and negative behaviors of other individuals is, "Well, you can't expect much from so-and-so, you know how he is..." In this strategy, the employee focuses on the personality problems of others as the reasons for his or her own decreased performance or inability to accomplish required tasks. |
| Confrontation | Certain personality types are more argumentative by nature, and even routine operations and tasks may be met with confrontation and disagreement, wasting time, and disrupting group harmony. |
| Criticism | A morale problem is created when an individual employee is criticized over a long period of time. This may result in a defensive nature of that employee and counter-criticizing those who criticize him or her. |
| Erosion of performance | General negative feelings in the workplace over time leads to decreased worker performance. This may lead to employees asking for a departmental transfer or searching for another workplace. |
| Regression | Continued erosion of performance leads to regression of the department or organization. Regression must be corrected, especially in the context of the modern health u-care industry, where there is a push for progressive changes, improved employee productivity, and improved quality of services. |

Adapted from Lombardi, D. N. (1993). *Handbook for the new health care manager.* Chicago: American Hospital.

Table 7-10

## *Strategies for Coping With Conflict*

| STRATEGY | DESCRIPTION |
|---|---|
| Withdrawal or avoidance | Avoiding a conflict-producing situation is appropriate when it is not the employee's problem, when there is nothing they can do about it, when it is not worth the effort, or when potential intervention may outweigh the benefits of resolution. |
| Smoothing or surrender | Smoothing is a strategy of avoiding the conflict by focusing on the positives instead of confronting the situation. This can be frustrating when employees are passive and perceived as the "good guy" by not intervening. Nonassertive employees often yield to the strategy of surrendering. Surrendering is appropriate when the other party is correct, the employee has little chance to win and wants harmony, or losing a small issue would mean a bigger win in the future. |
| Forcing or fighting | This aggressive strategy is used when an employee hopes to meet his or her goal at all costs; winning is achievement and losing is perceived as lowering in status. This tactic is necessary when a quick action is necessary (e.g., sexual harassment, violating safety regulations). However, it is possible that opponents will return for a retaliation at a later time in the future. |
| Compromising | This is a partial-win strategy in which middle ground is achieved and all parties feel comfortable. The negative limitation of this strategy is that neither party agrees on a equitable solution, and the focus is on settling for less on both sides. Compromising is appropriate when goals are incompatible, a temporary settlement is needed, and when discussions have not progressed. |
| Collaboration or collaborative confrontation | Collaboration is a win-win approach that builds positive and healthy relationships through resolving problems. Problems are resolved through open discussion, which leads to improved outcomes and results. Although generally this is the best strategy, a negative aspect of collaboration includes delayed decisions, which may lead to increased frustration over time. Collaborative confrontation is the strategy of directly dealing with the conflict-producing situation through a means of analyzing the situation and problem solving. |

Adapted from McConnell, C. R. (Ed.). (1993). *The healthcare supervisor: Effective communication*. Gaithersburg, MD: Aspen; and Umiker, W. (1998). *Management skills for the new health care supervisor* (3rd Ed.). Gaithersburg, MD: Aspen.

Table 7-11

## *Strategies for Preparing for a Confrontation*

| Strategy | Description |
|---|---|
| Visualize success | Practice success imagery by visualizing a successful confrontation. Visualize in your mind your body language, tone of voice, and your articulation of words. |
| Internalize self-affirmations | Adjust your self-talk by converting negative self-perceptions into positive thoughts. In our subconscious minds, we have a constant inner dialogue. Focus on the positive thoughts and self-affirmations by substituting "I'll try" thoughts (e.g., "I'll try to be in control next time") with "I am" or "I will" statements (e.g., "I am in control," "I will stand up for myself"). |
| Role-play | Rehearse your dialogue and anticipate the encounter by predicting the issues that will be addressed in the confrontation. Role-play scenarios with a close friend or confidant. Practice in front of the mirror. Your performance can always be improved. |

Adapted from Umiker, W. (1998). *Management skills for the new health care supervisor* (3rd Ed.). Gaithersburg, MD: Aspen.

- Emphasize the present and future, not the past. Focus on the problem and not the person. Clarify both the other person's viewpoints and your own.
- Be assertive and not aggressive. Use "I" statements by owning the problem (e.g., "I feel that…," "I am concerned that…"). Avoid the word "you," as it has an attacking connotation. Avoid sarcastic comments.
- Maintain a calm body language and keep eye contact.
- End on a positive note by thanking the person for resolving the issue with you. (Umiker, 1998)

The result of a conflict resolution through confrontation is variable, as there is never one answer, process, or solution to a conflict. However, confrontations are often not as bad as anticipated. Often times, if an issue is resolved through a conflict resolution process, the relationship with a colleague is strengthened. Effective conflict resolution, similar to a negotiation, requires preparation and practice, and can be a meaningful process to the occupational therapy practitioner. Although conflict in a workplace is inevitable, disagreements can be positive and healthy as long as they can result in a collaborative and win-win outcome for both sides of the issue.

# Appropriate Technology Use

As we move further into the digital 21st century, OT practitioners and students are required to demonstrate computer proficiency for a variety of purposes, including billing and documenting for services, typing reports and performance reviews, and communication.

Through the use of electronic mail (e-mail), instant messaging, and the Internet, practitioners are able to stay connected with colleagues on a departmental level, and even on a global level through a rapid and relatively cost-effective means. However, with the advent and increasingly popularity of e-mail come the strict guidelines of computer usage. Employees are finding themselves using the Internet for nonwork-related purposes in the workplace, which potentially decreases employee productivity.

E-mail is still considered a relatively impersonal means of communication compared to the telephone. However, health care facilities are now implementing network meetings via individual intranets and the Internet, so that people can communicate simply by sitting in front of a camera and microphone—both peripheral components to the computer system. Thus, people are able to verbally communicate with each other and observe nonverbal language (i.e., gestures, eye contact, appearance on the computer monitor) face-to-face, but without physically being in the same room. The advantages of computer technology are the flexibility, cost-effectiveness, and timesaving means of communication.

For practitioners less knowledgeable in the domain of computer technology and the Internet, many businesses and corporations have classes and workshops solely for teaching basic computer technology and Internet usage. Like any verbal communication strategies discussed in this chapter, Internet proficiency requires constant usage and practice.

## Documentation and its Implications

In the context of communication, documentation is a necessary component of the occupational therapy practitioner. With the emphasis on cost-effectiveness and quality of services of today's health care industry, quality documentation is essential.

Documentation should be clear and concise, and always include the date and relevant quantitative data (e.g., time, money, percentages, patient identification number). Depending on the type of documentation (e.g., initial evaluation, progress note, discharge summary), documents should be written in a timely manner within the guidelines of the department. Emphasis should be on content quality of the document. Professional language should be used; the use of subjective and biased language without evidence should be avoided. The end of all professional documents should contain the signature with the appropriate credentials of the practitioner. Communicating effectively through clear and effective documentation remains a critical consideration in ethical, legal, and reimbursement matters.

## Conclusion

Beginning from the first day on the job, the OT practitioner should initiate establishment of a policy for open verbal communication, honest and direct dialogue, and constructive feedback with all colleagues (i.e., fellow practitioners, supervisors, other team members) for a successful performance in the modern healthcare industry. Consider the quote by Daniel W. Davenport, "The greatest problem in communication is the illusion that it has been accomplished." In the context of this chapter, this quote implies that communication is a continuous and ongoing process for the occupational therapy practitioner. Communication can always be improved with the consideration of all the contextual factors. The occupational therapy practitioner needs to examine the viewpoints and perceptions of the other person (i.e., manager, occupational therapist, occupational therapy assistant, and volunteer) and gauge their level of understanding, in order to engage in effective verbal communication. The strategies discussed in this chapter should begin to assist and guide the OT practitioner in developing his or her own personal, meaningful, and purposeful leadership skills for teamwork building and supervision success in the health care arena.

## CASE STUDY

*Lyndon, a certified occupational therapy assistant (COTA), was a new employee at an inpatient rehabilitation center with a full case load. He had only worked in the rehabilitation department for a few months and was still learning departmental policy and regulations.*

*Lyndon's wife, who had a baby 6 months ago, had just won tickets to a once-in-a-lifetime family vacation to Hawaii for 1 week at the end of the month. Lyndon, upon hearing the good news from his wife, immediately approached his supervisor and requested vacation time at the end of the month. Because the rehabilitation department was currently going through a process of restructuring and financial difficulties, his supervisor balked at his request for vacation time. As a last attempt, Lyndon proceeded to ask if there was anything he could do to receive the vacation time. Because the supervisor needed to prepare for an interdepartmental meeting in the next 10 minutes, the supervisor hastily answered, "No, I'm sorry. Maybe next time."*

*Although feeling dejected after leaving the supervisor's office, Lyndon was determined to find a win-win solution in order to get the vacation time on such short notice. Typically, Lyndon tended to give in during a confrontation, however, he decided that this opportunity was too important to pass up. Because he was unsure of what to say, in terms of articulation of words, and was afraid to overstep his boundaries, he practiced his assertiveness and gained confidence through role-play scenarios with his wife at home. Lyndon also remembered that he was a team player in the department and had the personal right to express his opinions, without violating the rights of other team members.*

*In order to convince his supervisor for vacation time, Lyndon decided to implement a negotiation strategy. In preparing for the negotiation, Lyndon wrote down his possible options in writing. He considered the supervisor's point of view and came to the conclusion that the supervisor would identify granting vacation times as a problem of a financial nature. Also, there would be a difficulty in finding a replacement when Lyndon was on vacation. Therefore, Lyndon focused his options on willing to work overtime, working weekend hours, or working on holidays. After writing his options down on paper, he collected all relevant workplace data, such as holiday dates and other COTA weekend schedules. Lyndon also asked collaborated with other COTA's for their willingness to fill his position for that week in exchange for working their holiday hours. He also decided to bring a calendar for visual presentation and organization ease. Lastly, Lyndon decided the best time to meet his supervisor in order to present his ideas by setting up an office appointment.*

*During the negotiation in his supervisor's office, Lyndon clarified his interest in a week-long vacation time at the end of the month. They both agreed to focus solely on the issue of vacation time and both wanted a win-win outcome. The supervisor presented the problems of financial difficulty, tight scheduling for the rest of the month, and finding a replacement for Lyndon during that week. Lyndon then proceeded to describe his written options, using the calendar as a visual medium. The supervisor rejected his ideas of working overtime, due to not having the extra funds to pay for overtime work.*

*continued*

## CASE STUDY (CONTINUED)

*After proposing to work on more weekend assignments in the next 2 months, in addition to finding COTA replacements for that week, the supervisor agrees with the proposal. Lyndon ended the negotiation by thanking his supervisor for the opportunity of working through this situation. The supervisor responded by telling him that he was impressed with the amount of work in preparation to resolve this issue and asked Lyndon if he wanted to be in charge of weekly COTA scheduling for the department. Seeing this as a beneficial opportunity to improve as a team player in the department, Lyndon readily agreed.*

*Lyndon was able vacation with his family for a week in Hawaii. The supervisor found a responsible employee to handle weekly COTA scheduling. Outcome: Both of them won.*

# References

American Occupational Therapy Association. (1996). *The occupational therapy manager.* Bethesda, MD: Author.

Cherniss, C. (2000, April). *Emotional intelligence: what it is and why it matters.* Paper presented at the annual meeting of the Society for Industrial and Organizational Psychology, New Orleans, LA. Retrieved August 29, 2002, from www.eiconsortium.org

Fisher, R., Ury, W., & Patton, B. (1991). *Getting to yes: Negotiating agreement without giving in* (2nd ed.). Boston: Houghton Mifflin.

Goleman, D. (1998). *Working with emotional intelligence.* New York: Bantam Books.

Lombardi, D. N. (1993). *Handbook for the new health care manager.* Chicago: American Hospital.

McConnell, C. R. (Ed.). (1993). *The healthcare supervisor: Effective communication.* Gaithersburg, MD: Aspen.

Metzger, N. (1982). *The health care supervisor's handbook* (2nd Ed.). Rockville, MD: Aspen.

Munn, H. E., & Metzger, N. (1981). *Effective communication in health care.* Rockville, MD: Aspen.

Umiker, W. (1998). *Management skills for the new health care supervisor* (3rd Ed.). Gaithersburg, MD: Aspen.

# CONTINUOUS QUALITY IMPROVEMENT

*Jennifer Kaldenberg, MSA, OTR/L, CLVT*

## Introduction

In an environment of constant change, cost containment, mergers, and managed health care, professionals must strive to provide quality care. Examining efficiency, effectiveness, and adherence to standards of quality management (QM) in health care is a systematic process for evaluating health care services (JCAHO, 1996). Efficiency refers to services that are both cost effective and timely in its delivery. Services must be effective in achieving set objectives or outcomes for care. Quality management programs are designed to measure and assess performance to ensure adherence to pre-established standards. These standards are established by state, federal, and accreditory organizations such as the Joint Commission on Accreditation of Healthcare Organizations (JCAHO). Hospitals and other health care facilities refer to this process in many terms: continuous quality improvement, total quality management, quality assurance, and performance improvement. The processes of quality assurance, quality improvement/assessment, and performance are all methods of assessment, yet vary in motivation (external vs. internal), focus (problem based vs. quality processes), delegation (departmentally vs. interdepartmentally), and outcomes (hiding problems vs. improvement) (Jacobs & Logigian, 1994). Refer to Table 8–1.

There are many methods for evaluating quality such as clinical audits, peer reviews, and accreditation. Clinical audits refer to a group of peers working collectively to review case records for adherence to established standards, pre-established by the peer group. Peer review is a type of record review based on criteria established by the individual department, for what is determined to be quality care (JCAHO, 1996; Rakich, Logest, & Darr, 1992). Maslin (1993, p. 177) states: "Common to both peer review and clinical audit procedures is the term *process criteria*, referring to the activities or procedures undertaken as part of good patient care." Accreditation is sought by

Table 8-1

## Differences Between Quality Assurance, Quality Assessment Improvement, and Performance Improvement

| QUALITY ASSURANCE | QUALITY ASSESSMENT IMPROVEMENT | PERFORMANCE IMPROVEMENT |
|---|---|---|
| Externally driven | Internally motivated | Internally and externally motivated |
| Self-oriented | Customer driven | Customer/data driven |
| Vertical | Horizontal | Organization-wide |
| Delegated to a few | Embraced by all | Embraced by all |
| Focused on people | Focused on processes | Focused on processes, systems, and functions |
| Hiding problems | Seeking problems | Seeking opportunities for improvement; utilizes benchmarking or comparative data |
| Seeks endpoints | Has no endpoints | Has no endpoints |

many hospitals and health care organizations as proof of providing services that meet established minimum standards for Medicare reimbursement (Jacobs & Logigian, 1994; JCAHO, 1997). When performance fails to meet these standards, the organization must assess the performance and attempt to improve the areas of deficit. Changes can occur organizationally, departmentally, or individually. When discussing quality management, we must not only look to the organization, but to each individual occupational therapy (OT) practitioner providing the services.

In this chapter, we will discuss JCAHO's QM program and then further examine the practitioner's role in ensuring quality occupational therapy services.

# Skills You Will Apply

## Communication

Effective communication is necessary in organizing, implementing, and reporting quality management activities. The COTA who participates in this aspect of clinical management will share information with colleagues who are also involved in the study, with the head of the quality management study team, and possibly with facility administration.

## Management Skills

The tasks of management are frequently a part of a quality management study. Therefore, knowledge of their procedures and purpose will be of benefit to the COTA who participates in quality management activities.

## Leadership

The COTA is encouraged to assume a leadership role by noting areas in practice that could benefit from quality monitoring.

## Ethics and Credentialing

Quality management activities are frequently a requirement of accrediting bodies and state regulatory boards. Assessing and improving the quality of care to the patients and clients we serve is also an ethical responsibility.

## Change Management

Results of quality management activities provide a sound basis for change, improvement, and growth.

# JCAHO

JCAHO is a private organization developed to survey hospitals, mental health care, home care, ambulatory care, and long-term care facilities. These facilities are evaluated based on standards established by committees comprised of peer experts within the Joint Commission. JCAHO (1997, p. 5) states that its mission is "to improve the quality of care provided to the public through the provision of health care accreditation and related services that support performance improvement in health care organizations."

Most health care organizations in the United States seek accreditation from JCAHO in order to prove that they meet the minimum standards necessary for Medicare reimbursement eligibility. Since the 1990s, JCAHO has placed greater emphasis on the evaluation of quality health care and has established a process for monitoring and evaluating quality standards, which has shown to be helpful in developing or improving QM programs (JCAHO, 1997).

## JCAHO's 10-Step Process

The 10-step process established by JCAHO provides the necessary steps for monitoring and evaluating quality standards (Table 8–2). This is a comprehensive process designed to assess and improve the quality of patient care, staff performance, and interactions. The process may be completed departmentally or interdepartmentally, as increased emphasis has been placed on a collaborative or interdepartmental process. If we look at health care delivery in rehabilitation, it is not an individual effort but a team working together to maximize the patient's outcomes. If services are performed as a team, evaluation should also be collaborative. JCAHO (1996, p. 19) states "through collaboration it aligns the vision of the organization with the work and goals of the individuals responsible for the organizations success."

The first step is to "assign responsibility" for monitoring and evaluating the specific activities. Responsibility for the overall quality improvement process generally falls under the director of occupational therapy services, however it is important that the individuals responsible for the direct care also assist in the process. Because COTAs are highly involved with patient care, they are in a prime position to collect data for quality management purposes. The AOTA *Skills Mix Document—Guide to Role Performance* (AOTA, 1998) supports COTA involvement with all aspects of quality management activities under the direction of

Table 8-2

# *The Monitoring and Evaluation Process for Assessment and Improvement*

| | |
|---|---|
| Assign responsibility | The organization leaders oversee the design and foster and approach to continuously improve quality including the use of intradepartmental and extradepartmental activities. |
| Delineate the scope of care | The organization, as a whole or as a department, delineates its scope of care and service. |
| Identify important aspects | The organization, as a whole or as a department, identifies high-priority key functions, processes, activities, etc., to be monitored. |
| Identify indicators | Teams of experts, inter- or intradepartmental, identify indicators for the important aspects of care and service. Indicators pertaining to structures of care are no longer emphasized. |
| Establish evaluation triggers | Teams of experts establish the level, pattern, or trend in data for each indicator that will trigger intensive evaluation. Statistical methods are emphasized, as is the fact that thresholds are not the only way evaluation is triggered. |
| Collect and organize data | The data collection methodology often includes a means by which feedback from sources other than ongoing monitoring is used to indicate areas for evaluation and improvement. |
| Initiate evaluation | When thresholds are reached and when other feedback (e.g., patient reports) identifies other opportunities for improvement, leaders set priorities for evaluation and establish teams, which evaluate the patient care or service function in question. |
| Take action | Greater emphasis is placed on focusing actions on processes, especially the hands off between departments and services. |
| Assess effectiveness | A greater emphasis is placed on assuring that improvement is sustained over time. |
| Communicate results of the findings | Findings of those performing monitoring and evaluation are forwarded to the leaders and affected individuals and groups. |
| Other feedback | Receive surveys, comments, suggestions, and complaints. |

the OTR. The COTA's level of involvement will depend on years of experience, knowledge in a particular area of practice and setting, and service competency. Not only does the occupational therapy practitioner working directly with the patient have a greater understanding of the aspects of care, but he or she can also integrate the findings of the quality improvement process into future treatments (AOTA, 1998; Griffin, 1993).

The second step is to "delineate the scope of care," including the primary functions of the department, such as hours of operation, types of services provided, types of patients treated, and who is providing the care (Hinojosa et al., 1998). For example, the inpatient occupational therapy department for the rehabilitation unit provides care Monday through Sunday from 7:30 a.m. to 5:00 p.m. for all patients admitted to the rehabilitation unit. This is a 26-bed unit, patients are seen in the OT clinic for a wide variety of diagnoses, all having rehabilitative needs. The staff is comprised of three occupational therapists, two certified occupational therapy assistants, and an occupational therapy aide.

The third step is to "identify the important aspects of care," which includes the key functions, treatments, and processes that may be categorized as high-risk, high-volume, or problem-prone (Jacobs & Logigian, 1994). These important aspects of care are the ones most appropriately evaluated by quality management activities. High-risk activities include the various aspects of care that place patients at risk for serious consequences if care is not received, for example, bed and wheelchair positioning and upper and lower extremity splinting and orthotics, due to patients being at risk for contractures, edema, or skin breakdown. High-volume activities are those services that occur frequently within the department, such as patient education, patient assessment, and home safety education. Problem-prone care might include those aspects of care that are found to lack compliance with standards, for example timeliness and completeness of patient documentation or infection control.

In step four, "indicators are identified" for the important aspects of care to be monitored by the occupational therapy department. Indicators established should identify the desired activity and outcomes of care (AOTA, 1998). Refer to Table 8–3 for an example.

In step five, "thresholds are established for evaluation." In determining how each indicator will be measured, establishing the benchmark or target for expected performance of the function, process, or service provided by the department. For the indicator of falls prevention, a threshold of 95% was established. This means that of all the cases reviewed, a minimum of 95% of all patients received falls prevention education and that education was completed and thoroughly documented.

The next step is then to " monitor the important aspects of care by collecting and organizing the data for each indicator" (Rakich et al., 1992, p. 459). As seen in the example in Table 8–3, data collection can be completed through chart review, patient and physician surveys, attendance records, etc. In order to appropriately collect and organize the data, the department or organization must first determine what standards or criteria to utilize to determine adherence to the indicator. Once data is organized, indicators are evaluated. When thresholds are met, the department or organization may look for other areas for improvement or evaluation. If thresholds are not met, further evaluation is completed to determine possible causes. Possible causes can be developed into further indicators.

Once the data is collected, organized, and analyzed, the next step is to "take action," determining what actions need to take place in order to improve care. In the example of falls prevention education, if thresholds are not met, the department supervisors may decide to hold education sessions for all staff, outlining the importance of education and proper documentation. After implementation or action the department must assess the effectiveness of the action. This will determine if improvement may be maintained over time. This would be assessed by continued evaluation of the indicator in the following quarter.

Table 8-3

## Indicators and Thresholds

| INDICATOR | THRESHOLD | DATA COLLECTION METHOD | POSSIBLE CAUSES FOR THRESHOLDS NOT BEING MET |
|-----------|-----------|------------------------|----------------------------------------------|
| Falls prevention education was completed and thoroughly documented as evidenced by:<br>• Falls assessment<br>• Documentation of education and patient/family understanding | 95% | • Quarterly chart review of 30 records by the OT<br>• Reports to OT director and QM committee | • Short length of stay |
| Patients received 3 hours of therapy daily to include OT and PT and at times, SLP as documented in patient's chart | 95% | • Same as above | • Testing/procedures<br>• Illness<br>• Patient refusal |

The final step is "communicating the results of the findings." The information gathered will be shared with the occupational therapy department and quality management committee. The quality management committee is usually comprised of administrators, quality management personnel, and department coordinators. The director of occupational therapy services generally presents the results to the QM committee in writing and at quarterly meetings. The QM committee may make further recommendations for remediation. Departmental communication is essential in fostering team development and motivating staff members to maximize efficiency and effectiveness of treatment. Occupational therapy practitioners who are involved in the QM process will have increased understanding of the indicators and their potential effects on the patient, the department, and the organization (AOTA, 1998).

With a strong quality management program, departments and organizations will show improved efficiency with decreased cost, decreased waste and improved productivity, and improved effectiveness, with positive outcomes and patient satisfaction. Quality care should always be thought of as an ongoing process for the organization as a whole and for each individual working within the organization.

# Continuing Competence

When looking at quality care, the occupational therapy practitioner must look at the overall outcomes of patient treatment and their individual professional competence as an OT practitioner. Hinojosa, et al. (1998, pg. 4) defines continuing competence as "a dynamic multidimensional process in which the professional develops and maintains the knowledge, performance skills, interpersonal abilities, critical reasoning skills, and ethical reasoning skills necessary to continue in his or her evolving roles throughout a professional career." This process requires the occupational therapy practitioner to understand that this is a continuous process of improvement (Griffin, 1993).

The American Occupational Therapy Association (AOTA), the national organization for occupational therapy practitioners, is committed to assisting its members in keeping abreast to advancements in the profession and establishing standards that define quality services. The AOTA has established a council to address the issue of continued competence in occupational therapy, standards of which were adopted by the AOTA Representative Assembly in 1999. With financial and time constraints commonly experienced by many occupational therapy practitioners, the AOTA has developed continuing education (CE) articles, self-paced clinical courses, workshops on disk, and online courses to assist its members in meeting CE requirements and obtaining CE units (CEUs) to the resources to keep current in a growing profession.

Occupational therapy practitioners must maintain and demonstrate the appropriate knowledge and skill level for patient treatment in varied roles. Many state licensure boards require documentation of continuing education (refer to your state licensure laws) in order to maintain current licensure. These continuing education credits should be related to the occupational therapy practitioner's individual roles within the organization.

As of 2002, the National Board for Certification in Occupational Therapy (NBCOT) requires practitioners to accrue 36 hours of professional development units (PDUs) over a three-year period in order to maintain certification and to use the credentials COTA® or OTR®. The requirement is intended to complement state licensure terms. Of the 36 units, 50% (18 PDUs) must be directly related to the delivery of OT services (NBCOT, 2002a).

Continuing Education Units (CEUs) are converted to PDUs, based on a formula established by NBCOT. In addition, NBCOT offers a listing of a wide variety of professional activities that may be applied to PDUs (NBCOT, 2002b). Practitioners must keep records of their professional development activities. At re-certification time, NBCOT will randomly audit re-certification applicants for the required PDUs (NBCOT, 2002a).

Occupational therapy practitioners must be able to demonstrate appropriate communication, interpersonal abilities, and problem solving in order to maintain professional relations with patients, family members, peers, and other health care professionals. Being able to adapt in order to meet the needs of the patient, family, or health care professional will foster greater understanding and may improve overall treatment outcomes.

Lastly, occupational therapy practitioners must always adhere to the Code of Ethics established by the AOTA. This code guides our practice and allows occupational therapy practitioners to make appropriate decisions and actions. Each occupational therapy practitioner is responsible for his or her own ethical practice.

Given the rapid changes within the profession of occupational therapy and areas of technology, it becomes essential for occupational therapy practitioners to continuously update individual skills and knowledge level (Griffin, 1993; Punwar, 1998). As a new graduate or an advanced practitioner, it is important to have a professional development plan in order to compete in an ever-changing health care environment. The professional development plan enables the occupational therapy practitioner to assess his or her own strengths and weaknesses, develop goals and objectives to improve skills or knowledge, and identify possible resources to meet the goals (Griffin, 1993).

# Summary

Quality management is an ongoing process that includes administration, professionals, and consumers. The process is completed to ensure the highest quality care possible. To sustain quality, administration and professionals must communicate and actively participate in the quality management process. The 10-step process provided by JCAHO will assist in the development of a comprehensive quality management program to monitor and evaluate quality standards. Assessment of quality does not stop at the clinic or organization; each individual occupational therapy practitioner must strive to provide quality services and take the responsibility for their professional development. It is every practitioner's individual responsibility to provide quality and ethical care.

## CASE STUDY

The occupational therapy department in a 16-bed inpatient rehabilitation unit has developed a quality management program to review the following:
- Splinting schedules and adherence to the schedules by the staff
- Falls prevention education and carry-over of the information for the patients
- Treatment minutes

The department including the OT director, OTRs, and COTAs collected data and completed a chart review. Splinting schedules were to be placed in the chart and documented in the nursing daily sheets for adherence to the schedule. Falls prevention education was to be documented in the OT daily notes, including patient understanding and carry-over. Treatment documentation was to be documented in the daily notes and billing records for a minimum of 45 minutes, twice a day (BID). Goals were established as follows:
- Splinting schedules and adherence to the schedule were documented 95% of the time.
- Falls prevention education was completed and thoroughly documented with patient understanding 95% of the time.
- Patients received OT treatment in 45-minute sessions BID 95% of the time; if therapy was missed, thorough documentation was included for missed session 100% of the time.

Thresholds for splinting and falls prevention were met at 95%, while thresholds for treatment minutes were not met and achieved 85% compliance. The OT department held a meeting to discuss the results. The OT department has two full-time OTRs, two full-time OTAs, and an OT aide. Department hours are from 8 a.m. to 5 p.m. Monday through Saturday, and Sunday from 8 a.m. to noon.

Identify the 10-step process for monitoring and evaluating quality standards. Further discuss possible solutions to remedy the treatment minutes problem within the department.

# References

AOTA. (1998). *Skills mix resources—Guide to role performance*. Retrieved August 29, 2002, from http://www.aota.org/members/area2/docs/sectionb.pdf

Griffin, R. W. (1993). *Management*. (4th ed.). Boston: Houghton Mifflin.

Hinojosa, J., Bowen, R., et al. (1998, January). *Continuing competency task force report to the executive board*. Bethesda, MD: AOTA.

Jacobs, J. S., & Logigian, M. K. (Eds.). (1994). *Functions of a manager in occupational therapy* (Rev. ed.). Thorofare, NJ: SLACK Incorporated.

JCAHO. (1997). *Performance improvement in home care and hospice*. Oakbrook Terrance, IL: Author.

JCAHO. (1996). *Using performance improvement tools in home care and hospice organizations*. Oakbrook Terrace, IL: Author.

Maslin, Z. B. (1991). *Management in occupational therapy*. New York: Chapman & Hall.

National Board for Certification in Occupational Therapy. (2002a). *Certification renewal requirements approved by NBCOT Board of Directors*. Retrieved November 13, 2002, from www.nbcot.org/nbcot/scripts/news_and_events/press_detail_031902.asp

National Board for Certification in Occupational Therapy. (2002b). *New guidelines for certification renewal*. Retrieved November 13, 2002, from www.nbcot.org/nbcot/scripts/programs/new_guidelines.asp#5

Punwar, A. J. (1998). *Occupational therapy: Principles & practice*. Baltimore: Williams & Wilkins.

Rakich, J. S., Logest, B. B., & Darr, K. (1992). *Managing health services organizations* (3rd ed.). Baltimore: Health Professions Press.

# 9

# UTILIZING AND CONTRIBUTING TO RESEARCH

*Amy Solomon, OTR*

## Introduction

As the field of occupational therapy (OT) grows and health care becomes more complex and result-oriented, the need for substantiating our intervention processes grows. As we shall see in this chapter, there is an increasing demand by consumers, third-party payers, and the professional community for practice that is substantiated by empirical evidence. Ottenbacher (as cited in Deitz, 1998) emphasizes a need for research that validates occupational science and supports occupation as a viable method of therapeutic intervention. The Accreditation Council for Occupational Therapy Education (ACOTE) of the American Occupational Therapy Association (AOTA) includes in its guidelines for academic programs requirements related to learning to use and participate in research (AOTA, 1998a, 1998b).

The purpose of this chapter is to acquaint the reader with general concepts of research and to outline research process and methods to facilitate understanding and application of research studies to clinical practice.

## Skills You Will Apply

In developing and applying skills related to using research in practice, it will be helpful to understand how skills that have been discussed in previous chapters relate to the concepts presented here. Related skills include:

## Leadership

The forward-looking orientation of a leader lays a strong foundation for research. The practitioner who sees upcoming trends, asks relevant questions, and answers them with dependable information has the opportunity to add to the knowledge base of OT and as a result, contribute to shaping the profession.

## Ethics and Legalities

Providing the best care possible to patients and clients is an ethical responsibility of all OT practitioners. By having the ability to critically read research studies and use the information to remain current and knowledgeable of developments in the field, practitioners are supporting the ethical concept of beneficence as they offer current and sound services. In doing so, practitioners also reduce the risk of malpractice.

## Business Considerations

Later in this chapter, we will discuss the concept of *evidence-based practice*, which simply refers to using intervention techniques that are supported by current research. Third-party payers will reimburse for services that are so supported. By being aware of current research in the field, occupational therapy practitioners are able to offer reimbursable services, which add to revenue streams and support the business interests of their organization, as well as strengthen OT from a business perspective.

## Credentialing and Life-Long Learning

Another ethical responsibility of OT practitioners is that they remain current in their knowledge and to advance their professional development. Building one's knowledge base by studying or contributing to research is one method of ensuring one's professional growth and development. Specifically for the certified occupational therapy assistant (COTA), participating in research is one of the pathways to achieving the advanced practitioner credential.

# The Purpose of Research

Research is the systematic quest for and analysis of information and is conducted for the purpose of answering a specific question in a methodical manner. Research occurs in science, as in medical research; in the professions, as in determining an appropriate courses of action; in business, as in investigating a potential market; and for personal reasons, as when one researches a vacation destination. For our purposes, we will examine research in the scientific and professional sense.

Smith (as cited in Gliner & Morgan, 1997, p. 1) sees research as "disciplined inquiry." Gliner and Morgan (1997, p. 1) refer to research as "a systematic method of gathering information." *Systematic* suggests the manner in which information is procured and evaluated. Rather than obtaining data in random fashion, sound research practices require that specific data be acquired in a methodical manner and analyzed by standardized procedures. Systematic processes for collecting data include the manner in which research participants are selected and the way in which data are obtained. Systematic analysis involves the application of standards, agreed upon by the scientific community, to research data. These elements will be discussed in further detail throughout this chapter.

## The Significance of Research in Occupational Therapy

The need for research in occupational therapy has received increased attention in recent years. Progress in research has been somewhat slow in the field of occupational therapy (Robertson & Colburn, 1997).

As health care has changed, both from scientific and financial perspectives, the need for sound research has increased. Competition for markets and limited funding has compelled all professions to produce sound evidence that their services are effective and cost efficient. To this end, research in occupational therapy accomplishes the following:

- It provides credibility for the profession to the health care community and our patients or clients, as well as the general public
- It increases the knowledge and theory base within the profession
- It raises additional questions, which in turn, generate further research
- It adds to the security of OT in the health care arena as we can confirm the efficacy of OT intervention with sound research
- It aids in defining quality interventions and expands our repertoire of services to offer out patients and clients

# Evidence-Based Practice

Evidence-based practice (EBP) means that decisions regarding interventions are made using the best information available and that the care provided includes methods that are supported by current and reliable research (Law, 2001; University of Sheffield, School of Health and Related Research, 2001). In addition, EBP has implications for OT from ethical, legal, and financial perspectives.

The ethical premise of beneficence states that OT practitioners will provide the best care possible for individuals who seek their services. As knowledge in all areas expands at increasing rates, it becomes more critical that OT practitioners remain current in the profession's best practices. In doing so, one is providing the finest and most current care to patients and clients. Of course, not all techniques that are new and current are in the best interest of the people we serve. For this reason, practitioners must be able to discern reliable studies from those that are less sound. The ability to understand research allows the practitioner to make this distinction.

Another aspect of ethical practice supported by involvement with research is that of continuing professional development. Clearly, obtaining new knowledge supports life-long learning, and this is upheld by the ability to understand research articles. In addition, contributing to research activities is one of the activities that can contribute to fulfillment of the requirements for the advanced practitioner (AP) credential for the COTA. Achieving the AP credential is a powerful statement of a continuing education accomplishment.

In the event of a legal dispute, a practitioner may be required to defend the techniques used in treatment and to substantiate them in terms of their proven efficacy. Researched and validated clinical practices that are well documented can work in the favor of a practitioner who must justify their actions under legal challenge.

Third-party payers have an interest in practices that are supported by research. Generally, reimbursement is available for services that reflect best current practices and when there is evidence supporting their use (Robertson & Colburn, 1997). The profession would benefit from expanded outcome studies that validate through research, the services OT provides.

# The Role of the COTA in Research

All OT practitioners are required to be educated in research practices to some extent. The *Standards for an Accredited Educational Program for the Occupational Therapy Assistant* (AOTA, 1998b) state that the certified occupational therapy assistant must be educated in methods of research to enable them to:

- "Articulate the importance of professional literature for practice and the continued development of the profession" [Standard B.7.7.1]
- "Be able to use professional literature to make informed practice decisions in cooperation with the occupational therapist" [Standard B.7.7.2]
- "Know when and how to find and use informational resources, including appropriate literature within and outside of occupational therapy" [Standard B.7.7.2]

For the registered occupational therapist (OTR), AOTA (1998a) publishes additional requirements for research training, which include the ability to understand and critique research, understand and interpret basic statistics, develop basic research studies, and understand the process for presenting and publishing research, as well as for procuring grants.

To fulfill their educational requirements, a COTA must be able to read a research study or article and understand its implications for practice. Additionally, in working collaboratively with the OTR, the COTA may assist in the collection of data for a research study or participate in some other capacity as experience and expertise allow. Therefore, the COTA is expected to be able to read and understand research articles and responsibly participate in the research process.

COTAs are the practitioners who are in the most contact with patients and clients since they provide direct services. As such, they are in an excellent position to notice trends in interventions and to raise questions about their effectiveness, as well as collect data as they interact with clients and participate in practice activities on a daily basis. In doing so, COTAs are in a position to observe intervention strategies that are needed and effectual. This allows COTAs the opportunity to contribute to the outcome studies that are currently of such importance to the OT profession.

Crist et al. (1994) states that the role of the COTA in research is to assist in the collection of data and to contribute to the research process. Independently carrying out research requires an in-depth theoretical background in OT and the disciplines that support OT practice that is beyond the scope of OTA education. Consequently, AOTA does not endorse the COTA as a primary researcher. AOTA does emphasize the role of the COTA as a contributor to research and articulates the importance of all OT practitioners to be informed consumers of current research.

# Research Terminology

In order to understand a research article, one must have an understanding of the terminology commonly used in research studies. Table 9–1 defines basic research terms. The reader will see these terms in studies published in professional journals such as *The American Journal of Occupational Therapy* (AJOT), and in other publications. By understanding the basic terminology, the reader will be able to more accurately understand and use the information in research studies.

Table 9–1

## Research Terminology

| TERM | DEFINITION |
|---|---|
| Control group | The group of participants that does not receive or have the independent variable. |
| Data | Information that is gathered from participants and that will be analyzed to support or refute the hypothesis. |
| Dependent variable (DV) | The outcome or change that is expected as a result of the independent variable. |
| Experimental or Intervention group | The group of participants that receives or has the independent variable. |
| External validity | A statistical term that indicates the results obtained from the sample in the study can be generalized back to the population. |
| Extraneous or confounding variable | A variable that is not under consideration in the study, but that has the potential to influence its outcome. |
| Hypothesis | A statement, supported by educated deduction and reliable information, that predicts a relationship between variables or the outcome of an investigation (e.g., community mental health center clients with schizophrenia who receive daily OT services based on their individual needs will require less frequent hospitalization than those who do not receive OT services). |
| Independent variable | A variable that is thought to influence the outcome of the study. There are two types of independent variables. An *active independent* variable is one that is given to the participants and is applied, such as an intervention. An *attribute independent variable* is a pre-existing characteristic of the participants that is thought to have an influence on the outcome, such as gender. |
| Internal validity | A statistical term that indicates the dependent variable is a result of the independent variable. |
| Levels of variable | Variations on a category of variable. For example, a variable might be a history of CVA. Levels of this variable might be left CVA and right CVA. |
| Participants or subjects | The individuals who take part in the study. |
| Population | A group of people or objects that meet specified criteria relevant to the research question (e.g., in the study of clients with chronic schizophrenia mentioned above, all community mental health clients with schizophrenia make up the population). |

continued

Table 9-1 continued

### Research Terminology

| TERM | DEFINITION |
|------|-----------|
| Random selection | A method of selecting participants for a study that ensures each appropriate candidate has an equal chance of being selected. The goal of random selection is to minimize the chance that participants are selected based on a characteristic that could influence the study. Random selection maximizes the chance that a pool of subjects with diverse characteristics will be selected. |
| Reliability | The ability of a measure to achieve the same results over time. |
| Sample | A subgroup of the population, randomly selected so that it is representative of the population. |
| Significance | A term indicating that, statistically, the results of the study indicate that the independent variable, in all likelihood, is related to the dependent variable. |
| Validity | A statistical term that indicates the findings of the study are correct. |
| Variable | A characteristic of the participants. |

Adapted from Gliner, J. A., & Morgan, G. A. (1997). *Research design and analysis in applied settings.* Fort Collins, CO: Colorado State University; and Deitz, J. C. (1998). Quantitative research. In M.E. Neistadt & E. B. Crepeau (Eds.), *Willard and Spackman's occupational therapy* (9th ed., pp. 829-841). Philadelphia: Lippincott.

# The Ethics of Research

In the interest of human rights, certain ethical standards guide research activities. These standards are meant to safeguard the physical and psychological well-being of participants. There are also standards that apply specifically to the researcher's conduct and activity. Deitz and Crepeau (1998) summarize research ethics.

## Researcher Conduct

The researcher is expected to provide truthful and complete information to participants (informed consent—see below), as well as representing the content and results of the study accurately. Falsification and/or fabrication of results is considered misconduct. In addition, plagiarism is clearly unethical, as well as illegal.

## Informed Consent

Participants, or guardians of the participants in the study, must be provided, in writing, with a full account of what can be expected as a participant. Informed consent statements can include, but are not necessarily limited to, the risks and benefits of the study, the duration of and time commitments of the study, how study results are to be used, who may review the study and its results, and procedures of the study. A participant's signature on a standard form and maintained in the study files implies consent.

## *Human Subjects Review Committee or Internal Review Board*

Performing largely the same function under different names, these groups represent organizations or agencies from which participants may be selected. They are responsible for reviewing proposed research projects in the interest of their clients. A research proposal must be reviewed by the boards of every institution from which participants will be selected. The organization with which the researcher works can provide the steps necessary to submitting a proposal.

## *Rights of Participants*

Throughout the study, participants maintain the right to withdraw at any time without penalty, regardless of the effect on the study. Participants must be advised of this right during the informed consent process. In addition, they are entitled to any of the interventions that are part of the research (and to which they would otherwise be entitled) even if they withdraw from the study.

# Types of Research

Depending on the research question that is being asked, the goal of the research, and the type of data that is collected, different research formats are selected. The two broad categories we will explore in this chapter are quantitative research and qualitative research. This section will describe the different types of research most commonly used today and the general purpose that each serves.

## *Quantitative Research*

Quantitative research represents the conventional research traditionally found in professional research journals. It is characterized by the use of data that is measurable in concrete terms, such as numerical comparisons, test results, and occurrences of a specific behavior. Statistical analysis is utilized in this type of research, rendering results that can be counted and expressed in concrete terms and numbers. It tends to be reductionistic in nature (Deitz, 1998). Quantitative research requires that the researcher remain objective and personally uninvolved with the subjects and study, interpretations of data are value-free, and the results of quantitative research can be generalized across time and circumstance (provided one is generalizing to the population represented by the sample) (Gliner & Morgan, 1997).

Types of quantitative research include descriptive studies, correlational studies, experimental research, and single-subject design (Deitz, 1998). These are defined in Table 9–2.

### STEPS IN QUANTITATIVE RESEARCH

The steps in quantitative research are discussed subsequently and can be summarized as follows:

- A hypothesis is formulated based in observation and substantiated by fact. A literature review is completed to support the hypothesis
- A protocol is determined, including participant selection processes, informed consent procedures, and data collection and analysis methods
- The research proposal is reviewed by the appropriate human subjects review committee or internal review board (IRB)
- Participants are selected and informed consent procedures are implemented
- Study is carried out, per proposed protocol

Table 9-2

| TYPE OF QUANTITATIVE RESEARCH | DEFINITION | EXAMPLE |
|---|---|---|
| **Types of Quantitative Research** | | |
| Descriptive studies | Seeks information that answers a question about a specific group. | How many children who received OT services for attention deficit hyperactive disorder in elementary school continue to receive OT in secondary school? |
| Correlational research | Determines the extent to which two or more phenomena tend to occur at the same time. Does not imply causation. | Do people who are 6 months post-CVA report a decline in their ability to carry out IADL tasks? |
| Experimental research | Compares two or more variables; looks at the same time. | Is Splint X more effective than Splint Y in increasing ROM to the MCP joints following flexor tendon repair? |
| Single subject design | Focuses on one subject; follows that subject over time with repeated measurement of the same variable with and without intervention. | Does Subject A show improvement in socialization when daily OT groups are provided over a week's time? |

Adapted from Deitz, J. C. (1998). Quantitative research. In M.E. Neistadt & E. B. Crepeau (Eds.), *Willard and Spackman's occupational therapy* (9th ed., pp. 829-841). Philadelphia: Lippincott.

- Data is analyzed
- Results are written up and disseminated

Each of the steps is detailed in the following discussion.

### Formulating a Hypothesis

A hypothesis is an educated statement regarding the anticipated results of a study. It is generally based on one's observations and substantiated by one's knowledge base. It is a supposition that one makes about a relationship between variables, given a specific set of conditions. A research study is conducted for the purpose of supporting hypothesis by demonstrating a relationship, or showing that no relationship exists.

Case Study 1 provides an example of a hypothesis formed based on a COTA's observations in community mental health practice.

In the course of occupational therapy (and other professional) practice, questions arise regarding the efficacy of certain interventions and routines. This scenario also illustrates how a COTA is able to make observations during the course of providing services. The next step for this COTA would be to bring the question to the attention of her OT supervisor.

## CASE STUDY 1: THE FORMATION OF A HYPOTHESIS

*Sandy is a COTA working in a community mental health center. She works primarily with adult clients who have long-term mental illness. About half of the center's clients receive OT services in areas of self-care, homemaking skills, vocational training, or social skills training, depending on the client's individual needs and goals. At times, clients may be admitted to the in-patient unit as treatment needs indicate.*

*Sandy notices a trend for clients receiving OT services to function more effectively in the community and require less frequent hospitalizations than those clients not receiving OT. Based in her knowledge of occupational therapy intervention, Sandy knows that OT facilitates performance in cognitive, ADL, and social-emotional areas, and that these are primary areas of concern to clients with mental illness. She wonders if an OT program, geared specifically to the individual needs of clients, will significantly reduce the overall rate of hospitalization.*

*Accordingly, Sandy formulates the following hypothesis: "Clients who receive occupational therapy services, based on needs identified through individual evaluation, will demonstrate a less frequent hospitalization rate than those clients who do not receive services."*

*Note the following about this hypothesis:*

- *It is based in a clinical observation as well as an understanding of OT practice and what it can provide.*
- *It is a conjecture or "educated guess" about what will happen, given a certain set of conditions.*
- *It is worded in the positive.*

### Selecting Participants

Before selecting participants, or involving them in any way, a researcher must obtain the approval of the human subjects review committee or IRB. These may also have other names, such as human ethics committee, or others. Case Study 2 illustrates the planning of a research study and the submission of a proposal to the appropriate review boards.

Participants (also called "subjects") are the individuals who will be involved in the study and whose involvement will provide the data that will be analyzed. Selecting participants (or "sampling") for a study is the process of obtaining individuals who will participate in the research study. There are several considerations to make when selecting participants for a research study. First, it is necessary to consider where participants come from and whom they represent.

A population (as referred to in research terminology) refers to the entire group of individuals who have the potential to be appropriate participants in the study. The sample is the smaller group that the researcher will actually work with in the study (Deitz, 1998). For research results to be generalized to the larger group, the sample must be representative of the population (Gliner & Morgan, 1997). Using the example in Case Study 1, the population in this case is all adult community mental health center clients with schizophrenia and the sample is the group that will be used in this particular study.

## CASE STUDY 2: SUBMITTING FOR INTERNAL BOARD REVIEW

*Sandy approaches her OT supervisor, Jonathan, during their weekly supervision session, describing her observations and suggesting the possibility of a study. Her supervisor agrees that this would present an opportunity for both practitioners' professional development, benefit the clients, promote occupational therapy, and reflect well on the community mental health system.*

*In subsequent supervision sessions, they plan the study, including their hypothesis, reason for the study, possible risks and benefits, informed consent processes, methods of participant selection, intervention methods, data collection, timeframes, and reporting methods. They also complete a review of the literature to support their hypothesis. Although Jonathan guides the selection of theoretical background for the literature review, both Sandy and Jonathan locate and compile the information from pertinent OT and non-OT sources. They decide they will submit the study write-up to AJOT for possible publication as well as submit a proposal to present the paper at the AOTA National Conference.*

*Because the clients they will be working with are involved with both the community mental health center and the county hospital, Sandy and Jonathan contact both agencies to obtain the appropriate paperwork to submit their proposal. They do so to the IRBs of both agencies and include all of the information listed above. Both boards approve the study.*

*Sandy and Jonathan may now proceed with their plans.*

### Random Selection

Random selection occurs when all individuals in the population have an equal chance of being selected into the sample (Gliner & Morgan, 1997). There are several methods of achieving random selection, including generation of random numbers by computer or a random numbers table. It suffices here to note that random selection is intended to achieve a sample that is truly representative of the population (Gliner & Morgan, 1997). When the sample is truly reflective of the population, the study will likely have external validity, meaning that the results can accurately be generalized to the population. In applying a research study to one's practice, external validity of a study tells the practitioner that the results are likely to apply to clients or patients if they are part of the population.

There may be situations where true random selection is difficult to achieve due to constraints on the availability of participants. This situation does not preclude the applicability of the study results, as long as the issue is addressed in the study write-up. Case Study 3 continues our illustration of the research process with selection of participants for the study and procurement of their informed consent.

### Implementation of the Study

In this portion of a research study, the independent variable is applied to the intervention group and not to the control group. This phase of the study lasts a predetermined amount of time and participants receive the intervention as agreed to when providing informed consent. Case Study 4 continues our example.

## CASE STUDY 3: OBTAINING INFORMED CONSENT AND SELECTING PROGRAMS

*Now that the review boards have approved the study from a human rights perspective, Sandy and Jonathan are ready to begin. They also must follow through on informed consent procedures.*

*Participants are to be selected from clients with schizophrenia at the community mental health center who have not received OT services. Having previous OT intervention could be an extraneous or confounding variable in the study. From the clients not receiving OT services, an adequate number of participants are randomly selected. Half are randomly assigned to the intervention group that will receive the independent variable of OT intervention, and half to the control group, who will continue to receive no OT services.*

*Clients are informed of their rights, the procedures of the study, and its risks and benefits. As some of the clients have guardians because of the degree of their disability, the guardians are contacted to provide informed consent. All but one client give their consent, and the one client is excluded from the study. He is informed, however, that in the event OT services are found to be effective in reducing hospitalizations, he will still be eligible to receive services, as this is part of ethical research. The signed informed consent paperwork is maintained on file as part of the research records.*

## CASE STUDY 4: IMPLEMENTATION OF THE STUDY AND DATA ANALYSIS

*Sandy and Jonathan have decided that they will collect data over a 6-month period. Jonathan, as the OTR, assumes the responsibility of evaluating the clients prior to intervention to determine their individual needs. In addition, he will be primarily responsible for the theoretical aspects of the study, as he has the appropriate background to do so. Sandy, as the COTA, will structure treatment activities that are meaningful to the clients and will implement the intervention. She will maintain the records of each client's participation, as well as records related to frequency and duration of hospitalizations. Because she understands the use of professional literature, she will locate and recommend relevant research material as appropriate*

*At the end of the 6-month period, the data are compiled. Jonathan, with his more extensive education in research, will determine the appropriate statistical test(s) to analyze and interpret the data. Because Sandy is interested in research and is pursuing her advanced practitioner credential in mental health practice, she is learning the specific tests that Jonathan applies to the data and contributes her observations to the interpretations. In the teaching role of the supervisor, Jonathan discusses her observations and validates them as appropriate.*

*When the analysis is complete, the findings indicate significance at the $p < .05$ level. Jonathan and Sandy contact AOTA for editorial submission guidelines to follow through on their decision to publish their study.*

*Analysis and Interpretation of Data*

The analysis of data in a quantitative study consists of applying the appropriate statistical test to the data. The selection and application of statistical analysis requires training in statistics and research, and is included in master's level curriculum for OTRs. COTAs participate in the research process by providing intervention, collecting data, and maintaining records. Other participation may be appropriate, depending on individual experience. Case Study 4 illustrates OTR/COTA collaboration in the research process.

Although COTAs do not receive training in statistical analysis, knowing what certain statistical analyses accomplish when reading professional literature facilitates understanding. Some of the more commonly used statistical analyses utilized in quantitative research and that appear in journal articles include t-tests, ANOVA (analysis of variance), Pearson Correlation, multiple regression, factor analysis, and chi-square. The selection of statistical method is determined by such things as how many variables are present, how many levels of each variable exist, whether relationships are being assessed between two groups or between participants, and whether measurements are repeated or not (Gliner & Morgan, 1997).

The goal of any statistical analysis (in quantitative research) is to determine, statistically speaking, whether the results of the study are considered significant. In a research article, significance is noted as $p < .05$ or $p < .01$. Lower case "p" stands for "probability." The first example ($p < .05$) means that there is a less than 5% chance (probability) that the results of the study occurred by chance, and a 95% chance that the results were due to a relationship with the independent variable. In the second example, there is a less than 1% chance that the results occurred by chance, and a 99% chance that the independent variable was related to the results. In an article, this would be stated as, "significance was at the $p < .05$ level" or "significance was at the $p < .01$ level," respectively. In the world of quantitative research, results must be at the .05 or .01 level to be considered statistically significant.

If significant, the findings are considered by the scientific world to be supportive of the interventions that comprised the independent variable. The interventions supported in this manner are considered to be substantiated by research and contribute to evidence-based practice. When OT practice is supported by viable research, it can be justified to third-party payers, other disciplines, and the general public, thus enhancing the credibility of the profession and expanding options for the clients that we serve.

# Qualitative Research

If quantitative research is reductionistic, value-free, uses "hard" data such as numbers, states hypotheses, and can be consistently applied across time and circumstance, then qualitative research can be considered as its opposite. According to Crepeau and Deitz (1998, p. 842), the goal of qualitative research is to "explore the meaning and interpretation of experience" and to discover themes that "emerge" in the process.

Qualitative research is characterized by the following suppositions (Gliner and Morgan, 1997):

- There are multiple realities that depend on circumstances and conditions and that are changeable
- The researcher is an integral part of the study and interacts with the participants
- The goal of qualitative research is not so much to establish a truth that can be applied across time and circumstance, but rather, to generate hypotheses and questions

Table 9-3

## Types of Qualitative Research

| TYPE OF QUALITATIVE RESEARCH | DESCRIPTION |
|---|---|
| Ethnographic research | Describes the culture, points of view, and meanings of the people from that culture (Spradley, as cited in Crepeau & Deitz, 1998). |
| Phenomenological research | Strives to understand and explain the true-life experiences of people as they understand them. |
| Grounded theory | Develops theory from analysis of gathered data. |

Adapted from Crepeau, E. B., & Deitz, J. C. (1998). Qualitative research. In M.E. Neistadt & E. B. Crepeau (Eds.), *Willard and Spackman's occupational therapy* (9th ed., pp. 841-847). Philadelphia: Lippincott.

There are multiple reasons for different phenomena and one cannot determine a singular cause-and-effect. Rather, phenomena are "shaped" by numerous forces occurring simultaneously.

Qualitative research uses words versus numbers, and information sources include interviews, written correspondence and records, verbal accounts, and audio or video tapes that are analyzed (Crepeau & Deitz, 1998). From the analysis, common themes are identified, and hypotheses are formulated based on the themes.

### TYPES OF QUALITATIVE RESEARCH

As in quantitative research, there are various types of qualitative research: ethnographic, phenomenological, and grounded theory (Deitz, 1998). Table 9–3 defines each of the types.

Steps in qualitative research:
- An area of interest to the researcher is determined
- The same research ethics apply to qualitative research, and the proposal must pass review boards
- Participants are selected
- Data is gathered
- Data is analyzed for themes and generation of hypotheses
- Trustworthiness is established

#### An Area of Interest is Determined

In qualitative research, the researcher identifies an area that he or she would like to understand in greater depth. In qualitative research, no hypothesis is stated. Rather, the researcher goes into the situation open to discovering themes and formulating a hypothesis based on what is found.

#### Participants are Selected

Unlike quantitative research, where random selection of participants is desirable, participant selection in qualitative research focuses on different priorities. In qualitative research, participants are selected based on the researcher's perception of their ability to provide insight into their area of interest. This is known as purposive selection. Likewise, while an adequate numbers of participants is critical to the validity in quantitative research; they are not in qualitative, which can be done with relatively few (frequently under 10) participants. Case Study 5 explores determining an area of interest and selection of participants.

As in quantitative research, the proposed study must pass the human subjects/IRB review.

## CASE STUDY 5: DETERMINING AN INTEREST AREA AND SELECTING PARTICIPANTS

*Since the results of their study were significant, Sandy and Jonathan have become curious regarding exactly what it is about OT that contributes to decreased rates of hospitalization in their clients. They decide that the most effective way to learn this would be to hear directly from the clients themselves. They decide to implement a phenomenological study to generate some hypotheses on this topic.*

*Once again, Sandy and Jonathan prepare reports for the Human Subjects Committees of the two institutions that are involved with their clients. In the proposal, they have once again addressed topics such as selection processes, methods of data collection, and have submitted procedures for obtaining informed consent from the participants. Once again, the proposal passes the respective boards' reviews.*

*To select participants, Sandy and Jonathan decide on certain criteria that would support them in obtaining the information they are seeking. To achieve a series of perspectives on their topic, they make sure that their selection of clients represents a range of functional levels. While achieving a range of functional abilities, they also ensure that their selections include clients who are cognitively and emotionally able to participate in an interview situation. They select six clients for the study.*

### Data Gathering

Data gathering in the qualitative process differs significantly from that of quantitative research (Gliner & Morgan, 1997; Crepeau & Deitz, 1998; Lincoln & Guba, 1985). There is a variety of sources for data in qualitative research. Researchers may conduct interviews; review journals, diaries, and different types of documents; evaluate correspondence of various types; and make observations. The researcher selects the method of data gathering according to the method most appropriate to obtaining the information they seek.

In addition, the qualitative researcher generally maintains field notes that may contain accounts of their activities, their reactions, and other thoughts (Crepeau & Deitz, 1998). While this is not appropriate protocol for quantitative research, it is considered part of the process in the qualitative approach (Gliner & Morgan, 1997; Crepeau & Deitz, 1998; Lincoln & Guba, 1985). In this way, the researcher becomes an integral part of the qualitative research process. Crepeau and Deitz (1998) emphasize the importance of accurately recording quantitative data, as this becomes the basis for analysis. Case Study 6 continues our illustration of the qualitative process.

### Data Analysis

The goal of data analysis in qualitative research is to realize emerging themes from the information collected from participants (Gliner & Morgan, 1997; Crepeau & Deitz, 1998; Lincoln & Guba, 1985). Unlike quantitative research, which looks for causal relationships

## CASE STUDY 6: DATA GATHERING AND ANALYSIS

*Sandy and Jonathan have decided to use interviews of clients and aides who are present in occupational therapy groups, observation, and their own field notes. Together, they have crafted interview sequences using techniques such as open-ended questions that are directed at revealing the participant's point of view. Interviews with clients focus on their perceptions of occupational therapy intervention and the influence it has had on their daily function. With aides, the interview questions are directed at the aides' perceptions of client's daily function and changes that they have noticed. They have once again decided on a duration of 6 months for data collection.*

*The researchers are also sensitive to the role they themselves play in the qualitative process. Some of the outside influences that Sandy and Jonathan consider are the diagnostic implications of each of the clients, support systems in their lives, and cognitive and social-emotional performance. Both Sandy and Jonathan take part in data collection as part of their roles in the qualitative process. As the OTR with more extensive theoretical background, Jonathan will interpret the data, with input from Sandy.*

*To establish trustworthiness, Sandy and Jonathan employ the methods of prolonged engagement, peer debriefing, and triangulation. Their extended contact with the participants on a daily basis over the 6-month duration of the study supports prolonged engagement. In addition, the participants, as clients of the community mental health center, know both practitioners, which adds to participants' comfort level with the researchers.*

*To accomplish peer debriefing, Sandy and Jonathan have established communication with the director of the community mental health center, who is a licensed psychologist with extensive experience with this population. To gain an OT perspective from an outside source, they have periodic contact with an experienced OT practitioner in the community. With both of these individuals, Sandy and Jonathan discuss various aspects of the data and their impressions and interpretations to verify that they are consistent with theoretical concerns and current practice standards.*

*Triangulation occurs as Sandy and Jonathan compare information obtained from all sources and check it for consistency.*

between hard data, in qualitative approaches, the researched interprets and draws numerous conclusions from the data. Factors that one considers in the analysis of qualitative data include, but are not limited to, the influence of culture, researcher impressions, and influences of the social environment (Crepeau & Deitz, 1998). The box above exemplifies some of the considerations that our fictitious researchers will consider in their particular situation. The qualitative researcher attends to influences that are specific and relevant to their circumstances. Qualitative research is more adaptable and malleable than quantitative.

In considering all factors and influences, and the way in which they interact with the data, themes common across the data are revealed; from these, the researcher builds hypotheses.

### Establishing Trustworthiness

The trustworthiness of a qualitative study is, in some ways, comparable to validity in a quantitative study. Trustworthiness of a qualitative study represents its rigor and how dependable the reader perceives the study to be. Remembering that the goal of qualitative research is not to apply information across all settings, generalize information, or to estab-

Table 9-4

## Methods of Establishing Trustworthiness in Qualitative Research

| METHOD OF ESTABLISHING TRUSTWORTHINESS | DESCRIPTION |
|---|---|
| Prolonged engagement | The researcher remains involved in the field with participants long enough to gain a well-rounded view of their perspective and for the participant to become comfortable in the presence of the researcher. |
| Peer debriefing | The researcher checks impressions and findings with other individuals who are knowledgeable, but who do not have a vested interest in the study. |
| Member checking | The researcher verifies data with the participants of the study. |
| Triangulation | Data is collected from different sources and using different methods to ensure continuity and accuracy across data. |

Adapted from Crepeau, E. B., & Deitz, J. C. (1998). Qualitative research. In M.E. Neistadt & E. B. Crepeau (Eds.), *Willard and Spackman's occupational therapy* (9th ed., pp. 841-847). Philadelphia, PA: Lippincott.

lish relationships between variables, trustworthiness is established when there is truth value in the study, or when readers of the study find credibility in the data collection and can appreciate the experiences of the participants (Crepeau & Deitz, 1998). Truth value can be established by employing the methods of prolonged engagement, triangulation, peer debriefing, and member checking (Crepeau & Deitz). These methods are described in Table 9–4. Case Study 6 illustrates how these methods are employed in our imaginary study.

Qualitative research can contribute to evidence-based practice, as can quantitative research, when it follows these prescribed steps to produce credible results. Deitz & Crepeau (1998) suggest that qualitative research is especially applicable to occupational therapy because of its consideration of individual contexts and meanings.

## Other Types of Research

Two other types of research, one a combination of quantitative and qualitative, and community-based research (CBR) may also be of interest to the COTA.

Because of the nature of information obtained in some situations, elements of quantitative and qualitative research may be combined in the same study (Gliner & Morgan, 1997; Deitz & Crepeau, 1998). In combining these, the researcher must make a judgment regarding which method best evaluates the data they seek and provides the information they wish to provide (1998).

## COMMUNITY-BASED RESEARCH (CBR)

CBR is a method that engages community service agencies with academic institutions. In the CBR process, the community agency or organization poses a question that it may have, or specifies information that they would like to procure. The academic institution provides the human resources to implement the research. CBR has the capacity to address an unlimited number of research issues, and supports academic research priorities while benefiting community service agencies and the populations that they serve.

## READING A RESEARCH ARTICLE

When one reviews a professional journal, such as *AJOT*, one sees that the articles in it are divided into predictable sections. Each section contains specific information, and it is helpful in understanding research articles to know what each section contains. Table 9–5 summarizes the typical sections of a research article and the information that the reader will generally find in each.

# Summary

In this chapter, we have reviewed types of research and described the processes of the two major approaches to conducting research studies. We have compared quantitative and qualitative research, and provided examples of each process. A combination of these methods was briefly introduced, as was community-based research.

In addition, the structure of a research article has been described, outlining the content that one will generally find in the sections of a published study.

The purpose of this chapter has been to introduce the OTA student to the process of research in support of the ACOTE standards. These standards require that students achieve the ability to articulate the importance of research for professional development, to utilize research responsibly in practice, and to locate and utilize professional literature as needed. This also supports AOTA's role description of the COTA as one who contributes to the research process.

Table 9-5

## Parts of a Research Article

| SECTION OF ARTICLE | DESCRIPTION/INFORMATION INCLUDED |
| --- | --- |
| Abstract | A synopsis or overview of the study describing purpose, design, and a brief summary of the results. Depending on the stylistic guidelines being used, the length of the abstract is usually limited. |
| Introduction | States the purpose of the research study and what the researcher hopes to accomplish by engaging in the study. |
| Literature review | Summarizes current and relevant professional literature that relates to the research question at hand. |
| Methods | Describes how the research was accomplished, including four sections:<br>• *Participants*: A thorough description of the participants and the selection process.<br>• *Instrumentation*: The type of instruments and tests used.<br>• *Procedure*: Describes the study step-by-step, including items such as how participants are assigned to intervention or control groups and instructions that were given during the study.<br>• *Design*: Describes the independent and dependent variables and type of research design that was employed. |
| Results | Summarizes the analyses used and the findings of the study. |
| Discussion | Discusses implications of the study, including the relationship of results to the hypothesis, the themes uncovered (qualitative), any limitations of the study, or any factors that might have been extraneous or confounding variables, and possibilities for follow-up studies. |
| References | A listing of all sources of information and sources that supply background and supporting data for the study. References are listed according to the stylistic format of the journal publishing the article. |

Adapted from Gliner, J. A., & Morgan, G. A. (1997). *Research design and analysis in applied settings*. Fort Collins, CO: Colorado State University.

# References

American Occupational Therapy Association. (1998a). *Standards for an accredited educational program for the occupational therapist.* Bethesda, MD: Author.

American Occupational Therapy Association. (1998b). *Standards for an accredited educational program for the occupational therapy assistant.* Bethesda, MD: Author.

Crepeau, E. B., & Deitz, J. C. (1998a). Qualitative Research. In M.E. Neistadt & E. B. Crepeau (Eds.), *Willard and Spackman's occupational therapy* (9rd ed., pp. 841-847). Philadelphia: Lippincott.

Crist, P. A., Halom, J. A., Hinojosa, J., McPhee, S., Mitchell, M. M., Schell, B. A., et al. (1994). *Occupational therapy roles and career exploration and development: A companion guide to the occupational therapy roles document.* Bethesda, MD: AOTA.

Deitz, J. C. (1998). Quantitative Research. In M.E. Neistadt & E. B. Crepeau (Eds.), *Willard and Spackman's occupational therapy* (9th ed., pp. 829-841). Philadelphia: Lippincott.

Deitz, J. C., & Crepeau, E. B. (1998). Qualitative and Quantitative Research: Joint Contributors to the Knowledge Base in Occupational Therapy. In M.E. Neistadt, & E. B. Crepeau (Eds.), *Willard and Spackman's occupational therapy* (9th ed., pp. 847-851). Philadelphia: Lippincott.

Gliner, J. A., & Morgan, G. A. (1997). *Research design and analysis in applied settings.* Fort Collins, CO: Colorado State University.

Law, M. (n.d.). Evidence based practice: what can it mean for me? *OT Practice...online.* Retrieved June, 2001, from www.aota.org/featured/area2/ links/link16.asp.

Lincoln, Y. S., & Guba, E. G. (1985). *Naturalistic inquiry.* Newbury Park, CA: Sage.

Ottenbacher, K. (1998). Research note: research should document that occupation is an effective method of therapeutic intervention. In M. E. Neistadt & E. B. Crepeau (Eds.), *Willard and Spackman's occupational therapy* (9th ed.). Philadelphia: Lippincott.

Robertson, S. C., & Colburn, A. P. (1997). Everyday practice is the basis of research. *OT Practice, 2*(3), 30-35.

University of Sheffield, School of Health and Related Research (2001, June) *Definitions of evidence based practice.* Retrieved August 29, 2002, from http://www.she.ac.uk/~scharr/ir/def.html

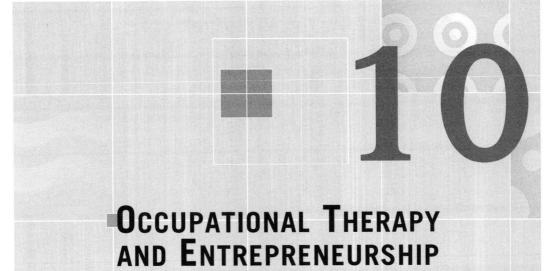

# Occupational Therapy and Entrepreneurship

*Amy Solomon, OTR*
*Karen Jacobs, EdD, OTR/L, CPE, FAOTA*

## Introduction

Think of a time that you or someone that you know had an idea or innovation that filled an identified need, promoted that idea or innovation, and perhaps succeeded in getting the idea or innovation, or a part of it, established as a solution. A situation such as this is *entrepreneurship*.

Entrepreneurship is the recognition of a problem or need, and filling that need by promoting a service, product, or idea. Called creativity, "thinking outside of the box," or perhaps any other number of terms, the skills of an entrepreneur can serve to identify areas of need and can offer creative solutions when they are needed the most.

Skills of entrepreneurship can be applied on a large scale in the larger, general health care environment, as when occupational therapists market themselves and the profession in new settings, as well as on a smaller scale, such as within a facility when the need for new programming is identified. The COTA, who is the primary intervention provider to clients and sees them consistently, is in a prime position to hear firsthand the concerns and needs of clients. This places the COTA in an excellent place to perceive clients' needs and promote programming relevant to those needs.

The purpose of this chapter is to explore the role that entrepreneurship plays in the ever-changing health care market and especially in the field of occupational therapy. The chapter covers entrepreneurship and promoting a program or service in a general way. The reader who is interested in program development is encouraged to explore resources in specific practice areas and to apply the concepts represented here to promoting their particular practice area.

# Skills You Will Apply

In developing and applying skills of entrepreneurship, it will be helpful to review and apply skills that have been discussed in previous chapters, also listed below.

## Leadership

Being entrepreneurial will require that you act as a leader by reading situations and responding to them in a certain manner. Effective entrepreneurship requires not only sound ideas and creativity, but a future-oriented attitude and strong judgment as well. Additionally, effective entrepreneurship will reflect ideas that are in response to the need of the profession, organizations, or the individuals involved. It will, in all likelihood, require one to learn from their mistakes. Learning to apply the principles identified in Chapter 1 will support the development of entrepreneurial skills.

## Ethics

A creative idea is appropriate insofar as it reflects ethical and legal guidelines. Reflecting the leader's dedication to ethics and "doing the right thing," an entrepreneur must exercise creativity and pursue ideas that, although creative, reflect ethical practice, and are within the parameters of professional boundaries.

## Change

Adaptive response to change is the hallmark of the entrepreneur. Understanding the change process and the ways in which people respond to change will help guide the entrepreneur in marketing change and innovation.

## Communication

In promoting a new idea, the ability to communicate, facilitate teamwork, and negotiate can influence the reception that an entrepreneur receives for an idea. Considering your audience and communicating with them in a manner that addresses their needs is critical to successful entrepreneurship.

# What is Entrepreneurship?

In her article "Emerging Practice Areas: Going Where No OT Practitioner Has Gone Before," Bethany Stancliff (1997) introduces us to occupational therapists who work in forensic hospitals, prisons, the home modification industry, shelters for the homeless, and within the industry as consultants. She introduces the article by describing the creative and innovative nature of occupational therapists, and how adept they are at finding new niches and practice arenas.

The practitioners that Stancliff describes are demonstrating the qualities of an entrepreneur. Allen (1999) describes the entrepreneur as someone who has the ability and executes the behavior of building an idea into a valuable enterprise. Other characteristics of entrepreneurs, according to Allen, include taking reasonable and calculated risks, planning strategically, and organizing resources and procedures into an innovative and successful business venture. Perhaps, more importantly, entrepreneurs have passion for what they do. They demonstrate a persistent quest for achievement, are independent, and are self-directed with an internal locus of control. Our goal in this chapter is to explore the role of the entrepreneur in the field of occupational therapy.

# Change

The world of occupational therapy is changing. Practitioners are competing for limited health care resources (Jacobs, 1998), and legislation such as the Balanced Budget Act (BBA) of 1997 has significantly impacted OT practice by limiting Medicare reimbursement for services. Jones and Carder (2000) emphasize the recent drive for COTAs to look outside traditional areas of OT practice secondary to the effects of reimbursement restrictions and changes in the OT job market. Many OT practitioners have shifted from facilities affected by the BBA to community-based practice, such as school systems. Others have promoted OT in new and innovative ways within settings that stand to benefit from the unique skills that occupational therapists offer. Yet, others have offered unique programming to meet new needs within more traditional settings.

Is change new to the field of OT? A review of significant milestones in the profession tells us that it is not. Gilkeson (1997, p. 172) cites the history of occupational therapy as "a tale of adaptation and entrepreneurship, of resourcefulness in response to changing times and needs." Her examples of entrepreneurs in OT include such leaders as Eleanor Clarke Slagle, William Rush Denton, Clare S. Spackman, Wilma West, Mary Reilly, and Anne Mosey. An examination of OT history and the contributions of these leaders in response to changing times illustrates entrepreneurship.

# Recognizing Opportunity

The individuals named above responded to change by offering something unique to meet a perceived need. Note also that individuals viewed as leaders in the field are also examples of entrepreneurs. Each of them recognized the potential and opportunity in change, and in doing so, moved the profession forward and fostered its growth. For these individuals, the perceived need served as an impetus for change. The need became an opportunity.

The current emphasis on community practice serves as an example of recognizing the opportunity in change. Occupational therapists' knowledge of performance areas, performance components, and the environment provide them with a strong foundation for assessing and adapting life in the community. As technology has enabled more people with disabilities to live in the community and competition for health care dollars has increased, cost-efficient intervention, such as community-based health care, has become a necessity. The skills and values of OT can very effectively meet these demands. While some view the changes in health care as foreboding, others see the opportunity to market OT in new "nontraditional" areas and move into these new areas. The section on leadership in Chapter 1 discusses leaders as agents of change.

Responding with innovative programming to needs that become apparent in one's own organization also entails a bit of entrepreneurship. Youngstrom (1999) defines five steps of program development:

- Formulating an idea, based on a recognized need
- Conducting a needs assessment to supply concrete data and confirm that a real need exists

- Provide a program description, complete with goals, population served, setting, outline of activities, and resource use
- Projecting start-up and operational costs, as well as anticipated revenues
- Devising an implementation plan, including preparation of the physical space, establishing a timeline for ordering supplies and equipment, preparing policies and procedures, and allocating staff

How does one make sense of change and organize oneself to move with it?

## Strategic Planning

Kotler and Clark (as cited in Strickland, 1996, p. 53) define strategic planning as "a managerial process of developing and maintaining a strategic fit between an organization's goals and resources and its changing market opportunities." In other words, planning strategically means that one looks to the future to determine where they might fit, and then implements a plan to move in that direction. Concepts of marketing fit with strategic planning. Both individuals and organizations can plan strategically for the future and market their ideas and services. Ethical, legal, political, economic, and social considerations are all part of strategic planning. The following sections illustrate the role of vision, mission, values, and goals in strategic planning and explain the situational analysis and the market analysis as methods for establishing a strategic plan.

The first step in strategic planning is to identify a need and market that your service or program can serve, as previously described by Youngstrom (1999). The next steps are:

- Set your ideal and goals through a vision and mission statement
- Identify your position through the performance of a self-evaluation (SWOT analysis)
- Complete a market analysis to determine the environment and circumstances in which you are offering your service
- Prepare a presentation tailored specifically for the target audience to promote your service or program

## Vision and Mission Statement

An organization's or program's vision is an ideal situation that the organization foresees. It represents an ideal for optimal performance of the organization (Strickland, 1996). The vision creates a picture of what the organization would ideally achieve in a perfect world. It is intended to be idealistic and extraordinary. An occupational therapist who envisions a program to develop the occupational performance of a specific population in need of service, and states an ideal state to achieve through OT intervention, is articulating a vision.

The organization's mission statement is a broad and general statement of what the organization or program intends to achieve. It lays a general framework for how the organization will operate, including where resources will be directed, the types of services that will be provided, and the methods that will be used to achieve this. Based on the vision, it paints a broad picture of the direction in which the organization will go to work toward achieving the vision (Strickland, 1996).

## EXAMPLE OF A VISION STATEMENT

*We envision the provision of service that:*
- *Enables individuals to engage in the occupational roles of their choice and perform related tasks in the environment of their choice*
- *Enhances the adaptation to living in the community*
- *Is sought by other professionals in efforts to achieve the above goals for their clients*
- *Is supported by legislation and funding sources*
- *Is cost-efficient*

## EXAMPLE OF A MISSION STATEMENT

*Our mission is to:*
- *Educate and demonstrate the appropriateness and efficacy of occupational therapy (OT) services to a variety of community settings*
- *Provide OT services to a variety of community settings, directed at their specific needs and goals*
- *Facilitate individual role and task performance in a variety of community environments*

# The SWOT Analysis

The acronym SWOT stands for "Strengths," "Weaknesses," "Opportunities," and "Threats." By evaluating these elements in one's environment, a comprehensive picture of the factors one must consider is achieved. Below we define each of these elements:

- *Strengths (S)*: Characteristics of the organization that enhance its position. Examples might include, but are not limited to, a strong financial basis, a relevant skill base, or strong support.
- *Weaknesses (W)*: Characteristics of the organization that may weaken its position. Examples include, but, are not limited to, the reverse of those listed under "strengths."
- *Opportunities (O)*: Niches where there is fit between the organization's strengths, the services it offers, and identified needs in the market. For example, if there is a need for a cost-efficient way to maintain older adults in the home, an opportunity exists for someone to create a means of providing that service.
- *Threats (T)*: Elements in the market that can interfere with or deter an organization from meeting its goals. Although they will not necessarily prevent goal achievement, being aware of threats enables an organization to prepare to meet them and strengthen pertinent areas. For example, if a competing group offers a similar but less effective service that is less costly, an organization can promote the benefits that they offer and emphasize their cost effectiveness in comparison to the other group.

To accomplish a SWOT analysis, Jacobs and Logigian (1999) suggest performing a self-evaluation that considers areas such as staff qualifications and expertise; physical attributes of your program, such as size, location, setting, and available equipment; financial resources; and administrative support. Each area is evaluated to determine whether it will strengthen or weaken, be an opportunity, or pose a threat to your goal. In reviewing the example in Table 10–1, one might draw the following conclusions:

- OTs have a well-rounded background and numerous strengths that can be beneficial to consumers in the community; however, this is not well understood by the general public.
- Self-advocacy has not, historically, been a strong point for OT practitioners, although AOTA has increased its marketing efforts in recent years and strongly supports and promotes community practice.
- There is an increasing number of people in the community who require or desire services, and legislation supports this. Community-based care is a cost-effective approach to intervention, yet this is (again) poorly understood by the general public.
- Other disciplines may be perceived as being able to do the "same thing" as OT personnel, and for less money.

By reviewing these points, one is able to recognize aspects of one's position that can be used as a marketing tool, as well as identify potential areas of deficiency and allow for planning to address them.

# The Market Analysis

Other factors that may be considered include competing programs, the political and financial environments, and the demographic factors of your target market. The goal of completing a market analysis is to gain a sense of the environment in which you plan to market or promote your service or program. A market analysis will inform you of your target audience's needs, the services they provide, where "gaps" in service may exist, as well as the political and financial issues that could ultimately affect your program or service. Because you have completed your SWOT analysis, you have a sense of how your strengths can support market needs and what potential pitfalls you need to be prepared to address.

## The Target Audience and Needs Assessment

The target audience is the primary group to whom you wish to promote your service or program. The target audience may be any individual or group that may be a potential stakeholder in the program you are marketing. Many times, the target audience includes decision-makers and funding sources, and marketing to them becomes critical to your success. Examples of possible target audiences include, but are not limited to, physicians, a board of directors of a nonprofit organization, the owner or chief executive officer (CEO) of a corporation, parents, administrators, clients, and others.

Each target audience will have its own goals, needs, and priorities, and they are most interested in how your proposed program or service can serve them in meeting those goals and priorities.

Table 10-1

## Example of a SWOT Analysis

| STRENGTHS | WEAKNESSES | OPPORTUNITIES | THREATS |
|---|---|---|---|
| OTs have an in-depth knowledge of performance in all areas. | OT is poorly understood by the community and general public. | There is an increasing number of people in the community who require services, due in part to shorter inpatient stays. | Other disciplines may be perceived as doing the "same thing." |
| OTs have an in-depth knowledge of adaptation for living in the community. | OTs have historically not been their own best advocates. | Community-based care is more cost-efficient than inpatient care, and OTs can support community-based interventions. | Funding for services may be limited. |
| OTs have an understanding of environmental demands and adaptations. | Many OT practitioners prefer to remain in the comfort zone of traditional medical practice. | Legislation, such as the ADA, offers OT a niche. | |
| Because of their medical backgrounds, OTs have an understanding of medical conditions and issues that should be addressed. | OTs may lack marketing and promotional strategies and funds. | The population ("baby boomers") is aging and value activity, which may represent a niche for OT. | |
| OT personnel have an understanding of advocacy and legal issues, such as those associated with the ADA. | | | |
| OT may reduce the need for more costly inpatient stays, as it has the potential to maintain an individual's function in the community. | | | |
| AOTA is a strong resource and support for community practice. | | | |

# Assessing Needs

To effectively understand the priorities of your target audience, the following questions may be asked:

- What services does the target audience provide?
- Are there additional services they would like to provide?
- What are their goals and priorities? In what areas do they wish to grow?
- How does your proposed service or program support what they are already doing?
- How does your proposed service or program fill their "gaps" and/or help them achieve their goals?
- What other services or programs are available that might compete with yours?
- What federal, state, and local legislation supports or otherwise affects provision of service?
- What financial and funding issues support or otherwise affect provision of service?
- Can your service or program address any additional areas?

Finding the answers to these questions requires some research and investigation. The Internet is an excellent source, as many organizations include their strategic goals, services offered, and other relevant information on their web sites. Informational interviews with key personnel can also be a source of data. Other sources may include professional organizations and library records.

In finding the answers to these questions (and any others that you feel are pertinent), one is able to determine the position of the target audience and decision-makers. Used in conjunction with the SWOT analysis (the determination of your position), a clear picture of a match (or lack thereof) between your service and the target audience can be determined. In evaluating these perspectives, a strategic communication to promote your service or program can be developed.

# Strategic Communication for Marketing

Occupational therapy personnel are not strangers to strategic communication. In working with patients, clients, and families, OTs employ techniques of listening—learning the patient's or client's situation and responding to their needs and goals—and, with the input of the patient, client, and family, construct an intervention plan and activities. Marketing is simply showing how your program, organization, or idea can fill a need or provide a needed service. Strategic communication, in terms of thinking a communication through and responding in a thoughtful manner, is similar to the thought that one puts into communicating with patients and clients.

Do consider that there are optimal times and methods for communicating in any situation. As with clients and their families, the environment and setting play a part in how a message is received. Likewise, when promoting an idea or proposal, it is necessary to consider:

- *The setting:* In your situation, where is the appropriate place to present your idea? Organizational culture and ritual will, in large part, determine this. The appropriate setting may be in a regular meeting, in a specially arranged meeting, or in an individual appointment. The content of your proposal and the relationships you have with colleagues may also influence your choice of setting. You will need to evaluate this, possibly with the help of a mentor or supervisor.

- *Timing*: Timing can be a critical factor in presenting a proposal. In doing your SWOT and market analyses, you will know the current priorities and needs of the audience. Select a time when other priorities are not foremost in the minds of decision-makers in order to ensure that your proposal receives full attention. If your audience is distracted by other issues that are currently more pressing, your proposal may not receive the consideration you would like. Be aware also of the amount of time that you have to complete your presentation, and stay within the allotted time.

- *Content*: Avoid the temptation to relate all the information that you have on your proposal and its background. Carefully select information that is relevant to promoting your plan in a manner that makes it attractive to the audience and gives them the idea that the information is sensible and feasible. Themes can be expanded on later and as additional information is requested. In the initial phases, it is best not to "overload" with too much information. Provide additional information as it can be processed.

- *Method of presentation*: In different organizations, acceptable methods of presentation may vary. Depending on your audience, the setting in which a proposal is made, and the traditions of the organization, a more or less formal presentation may be required. Know what the expectations are. Is a formal, computer-generated presentation most appropriate? Or is an open discussion more fitting to the organizational culture? Or is something in between these, such as a brief talk and flip chart most fitting? These are elements that will be determined individually, and may even vary depending on the proposal. Again, a mentor or supervisor can assist the beginning entrepreneur in making this decision.

## Listening

The basic elements of listening, as described in Chapter 6, form the foundation for any communication. When strategic communication is applied to promoting an idea, the following components are also critical.

O'Hair, Friedrich, and Shaver (1998, p. 104) define listening as "a voluntary process that goes beyond reacting to sounds and includes understanding, analyzing, evaluating, and responding." In strategic communication, these elements are critical. In presenting your program or idea, truly listening to and responding to the needs of the target audience can make the difference in whether your idea is accepted or not.

To accomplish these goals and truly "hear" what those needs are, consider the following:

- Remain focused on what your audience is saying. Avoid the tendency to become distracted by your own thoughts or by being preoccupied with concerns other than what the speaker is telling you.

- Be aware of how your perceptions color the way you hear others. Your experience influences the manner in which you comprehend other people and situations, and in order to effectively relate your plan or idea, it is necessary to determine your perceptions, know how they are affecting your listening and communication, and set them aside. It is to your advantage to understand the role and respond to the perceptions of the target audience versus your own.

- Understand the perceptions of the target audience. In some respects, by recognizing a need and paying attention to it, you have already done this to some extent. When presenting your plan or idea, it is also necessary to listen carefully to how your audience is perceiving you and what you have to say. It is equally important to respond in a manner that addresses their concerns and supports their interests.

- Employ the therapeutic use of self techniques that you have learned to use with clients and patients. Applying principles of developing empathy can assist you in understanding your target audience's perspective. Pay attention to nonverbal communication and the motivation of your audience. To discover these elements so that you may respond, ask open-ended questions.

## Processing What is Said

To a large extent, listening actively requires that you think about what is being said and that you respond thoughtfully in order to communicate effectively. To accomplish this, the following recommendations are helpful:

- Discern the needs and priorities of your audience. In order for the target audience to remain open to your idea or plan, you must demonstrate an understanding of their priorities and objectives.

- Think about the emotions behind what is being said, and consider how these affect how the audience perceives the issues being discussed.

- Consider how your proposal meets the practical priorities and emotional elements of your audience.

By actively thinking about and processing these elements as you listen, you will be able to formulate a more effective response and increase your chances of successfully promoting your idea.

## Responding

In formulating a response to questions or comments, it is (obviously) necessary to take into consideration all of the factors mentioned up to this point. The key factor to bear in mind is that any responses should be directed at meeting the needs of the target audience. How can your proposal support them in meeting their goals and priorities?

- *Benefits*: What benefits exist for the target audience? Does your proposal help them achieve a desired outcome? Does it help them deliver a service? Does it help them reach a desired population? These are only a few possible benefits for a target audience. It is your job to let them know how your proposal or idea will support them in accomplishing their goals.

- *Cost-effectiveness*: In today's economic climate, any proposal must be cost-effective. Your success in promoting your plan or idea will be directly linked to your ability to demonstrate its efficiency in terms of cost savings or generating a revenue stream. Supporting your proposal with well-researched figures strengthens your case.

- *Language*: In presenting your proposal or plan, be cognizant of the language that you choose. Be especially aware of words or expressions that could be interpreted as racist or sexist. Developing an awareness of the cultural and social expectations of the individuals in your audience will facilitate the acceptance that your plan receives.

- *Monitoring your emotions*: In presenting a plan or proposal, it is natural to have emotional attachment and personal investment in your idea and the work that you have put into it. Being passionate about your proposal is a positive thing! At the same time, it is important to remain objective and bear in mind that questions or objections that raised pursuant to your proposal are not directed at you personally, nor are they intended to undermine your idea. Hear them with an open mind, applying the concepts of listening discussed previously. Then, process what is being said and respond in a calm and objective manner, also using the principles listed in this chapter. The following steps may be helpful:
  1. Avoid taking a defensive stance. Remember that this is not a personal attack but a question about how the plan benefits the audience.
  2. Use reflection to clarify the point being made and the emotion behind it. If you have misinterpreted something, request clarification.

Communicate ethically and responsibly. Provide factual information, and if you are unsure of an answer, say so and offer to find the information. Follow through!

# Marketing and Promoting the Profession

Marketing is a process that involves developing and promoting a product or service that meets the specific needs of an identified consumer or consumer group (Pride & Ferrell, 1997; Palmer & Stull, 1991). To apply it to the concepts of entrepreneurship and promoting an idea, we may view marketing as promoting occupational therapy in the larger scheme of health care and the community. Using Stancliff's (1997) examples, these occupational therapy practitioners marketed the profession to new consumer groups. One may think of marketing and promoting the profession as applying the concepts of entrepreneurship on a larger scale.

In addition to identifying a need, and proposing programming to meet those needs, marketing also involves promotion, advertising, publicity, and cost control (Jacobs, 1998). One of the challenges that occupational therapy has historically faced as a profession is explaining our services in manner that promotes them in a variety of settings, while maintaining their uniqueness in the light of other services. Part of effective marketing—especially in new and emerging practice settings and in traditional settings—is explaining occupational therapy in a way that emphasizes how OT fits in a specific setting.

The details of the marketing process as described by Jacobs (1999) beyond the concepts of entrepreneurship addressed here are outside of the scope of this entry-level text. For the COTA who is interested in pursuing marketing, there are numerous resources in the literature. The AOTA is an excellent resource for marketing specific aspects of OT and the profession as a whole. The reader is also referred to the references listed at the conclusion of this chapter.

# Summary

Entrepreneurship is the process of recognizing a need, formulating a creative idea or solution in response to that need, and promoting it. Marketing is, in part, getting that idea or solution across to the target audience. Marketing may also be implemented on a larger scale and involves the study of additional strategies and concepts, which the reader is encouraged to research if their interests take them in that direction.

Our discussion of entrepreneurship identified the following components of promoting an idea or program:

- Identify a need or opportunity
- Develop a program or idea in response to the need
- Define your direction with a vision and mission statement
- Perform a SWOT analysis to define the specifics of your situation
- Perform a market analysis to define the specifics of the external environment
- Implement the principles of strategic communication to market your plan

# References

Allen, K. R. (1999). *Launching new ventures: An entrepreneurial approach* (2nd ed.). New York: Houghton Mifflin.

Gilkeson, G. E. (1997). *Occupational therapy leadership: Marketing yourself, your profession, and your organization.* Philadelphia: F. A. Davis.

Jacobs, K. (1998, November 5). The art of negotiation. *OT Week 12*(45), 10-11.

Jacobs, K., & Logigian, M. K. (1999). *Functions of a manager in occupational therapy* (3rd ed.). Thorofare, NJ: SLACK Incorporated.

Jones, R. A., & Carder, C. J. (2000). *Exploring non-traditional employment settings and strategies for OTAs.* Paper presented at the annual conference of the American Occupational Therapy Association, Seattle, WA.

O'Hair, D, Friedrich, G. W, & Shaver, L. D. (1998). *Strategic communication in business and the professions.* Boston: Houghton Mifflin.

Palmer, D., & Stull, W. A. (1991). *Principles of marketing* (2nd ed.). Cincinnati, OH: Southwestern.

Pride, W. M., & Ferrell, O. C. (1997). *Marketing: concepts and strategies* (10th ed.). Boston: Houghton Mifflin.

Stancliff, B. L. (1997). Emerging practice areas: Going where no OT has gone before... *OT Practice, 2*(7),16-32.

Strickland, L. R. (1996). Strategic planning. In AOTA (Ed.) *The occupational therapy manager* (pp. 51-61). Bethesda, MD: AOTA.

Youngstrom, M. J. (1999). Developing a mew occupational therapy program. In K. Jacobs & M. K. Logigian (Eds.) *Functions of a manager in occupational therapy* (3rd ed., pp. 129-142). Thorofare, NJ: SLACK Incorporated.

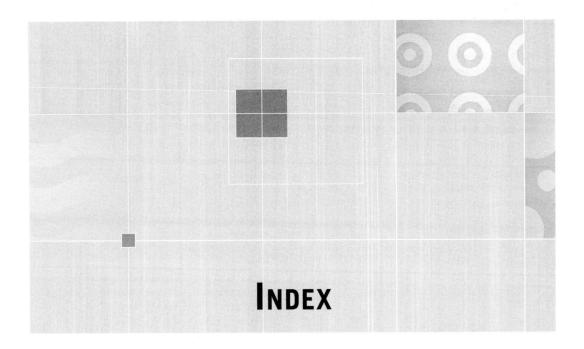

# INDEX